U.S.S. Red Rover

Civil War Hospital Ship

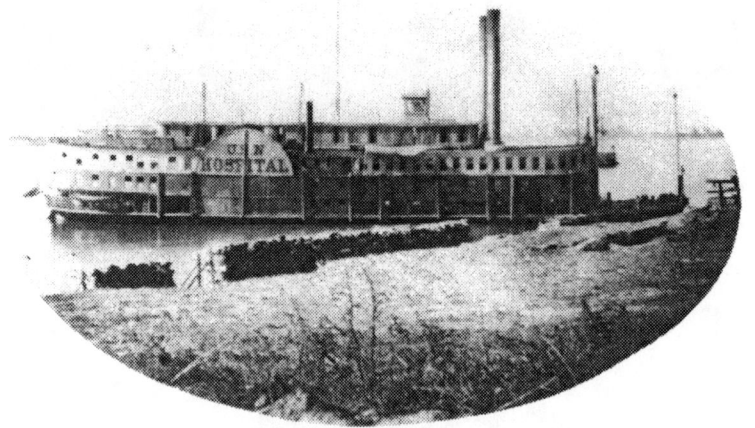

By
Wm. L. Dike

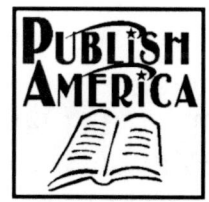

PublishAmerica

Baltimore

First printing

ISBN: 1-4137-1488-9

PUBLISHED BY PUBLISHAMERICA, LLLP

www.publishamerica.com

Baltimore

Printed in the United States of America

Dedicated to the women and men
who gave as sacrificially
as the combatants
through their caring
for the sick and wounded

HUMBLE AND BRIEF BEGINNINGS

Red Rover, the first hospital ship of the U.S. Navy, was built at Cape Girardeau, Missouri, in 1859. Her length was 256 feet and she had a draft of eight feet and a top speed of nine knots, which required the burning of thirty-seven and half bushels of coal per hour. She was built as a commercial sidewheel steamer, which, based on a postally used advertising envelope, was intended to ply the Mississippi River between New Orleans and Nashville. *Red Rover*'s commercial career was brief as she was purchased for use as a barracks or "accommodations" ship by the Confederate States of America on November 7, 1861.

In a Memorandum extract from his personal papers we read:

> John Julius Guthrie, lieutenant, commanding, C. S. Navy, was ordered to assume command of the steamer Red Rover, purchased at New Orleans, La., for $30,000, this day, November 7, 1861. Was ordered to proceed to Memphis, Tenn., November 25, 1861, or other place to meet the floating battery New Orleans. Joined her near Columbia, Ark., and arrived at Columbus, Ky., December 11, 1861.

The *New Orleans* had been commissioned at New Orleans October 14, 1861. Under the joint command of Lieutenant Guthrie both the floating battery *C.S.N. New Orleans* and *Red Rover* assisted the Confederate defense of Columbus, Kentucky. They then moved on to become a part of the Confederate's rather formidable force attempting to block the Federal Gunboat Flotilla at Island No. 10 in the Mississippi River, near New Madrid, Missouri. In early March, Lieutenant Guthrie was relieved by Lieutenant G. W. Averett and the latter was the commanding officer of both vessels when

Federal forces put Island No. 10 under siege.

Red Rover's third career commenced with the Federal bombardment of Island No. 10 on March 15, 1862. On March 25, 1862, Lieutenant Averett wrote to Confederate Flag Officer George N. Hollins, Commanding Naval Forces, Mississippi:

I am informed by Captain Huger that you desire to know my idea of affairs at this place. This is the eleventh day of the bombardment. I think the entire results may be stated at 2 killed and 7 wounded on shore. I believe we are stronger here to-day than when the enemy first appeared. The enemy's gunboats and mortar boats have not been within the effective range of the battery. I have fired one shot at a transport as an experiment for the range of one of my rifle guns. She changed her berth soon afterwards. On the evening of the 17th two fieldpieces fired three shots at the battery from the opposite bank, but a few well-directed shots drove them off and I have good reason to believe that one of the field carriages was broken and 2 men killed. On the following evening two more pieces were discovered coming down toward the same point, but they were driven off by the battery. before they fired a shot. The battery has fired altogether twenty-nine shots and shells. Some of these were fired to break up the enemy's signaling from the shore to their boats and to disperse squads of them who would occasionally show themselves together. The officers and soldiers of Captain O'Hara's Pelican Guards and of Captain Stubbs' company of the First Alabama Regiment have conducted themselves in a manner to satisfy me that they are men of determined gallantry and will make a fight worthy of the cause they are serving. The latter company has been under the charge of Lieutenant Stone and recently under that of Lieutenant Crockett. Captain Cooper's company from the Forty-sixth Tennessee Regiment was serving with me up to the 17th, when they were ordered away. This leaves me short of crews for two guns. I have repeatedly tried to get men for them, and orders have been given for captains to report their companies to me, but there seems to be the greatest objections to serving on board the battery, and I have for the present given up the hope of additional help from the army. Of the navy part of my command I can hardly speak too well. The officers and crew alike have evinced the best spirit and have done their duties well and faithfully. Mr. Gift remained with me six days after the acceptance of his resignation and by his vigilance and prompt execution of my orders, gave me much assistance. Acting Master Guthrie has been on leave till yesterday. Acting Master Erwin has unfortunately been sick during this interesting time. There have been no casualties on board the battery and the Red Rover. The battery has been struck by fragments of shells and severely jarred by their explosions under her and around her, but is unharmed. The Red Rover was cut through all her decks to her bottom by a piece of shell, which caused her to leak considerably, but not dangerously. She has not been our quarters since the enemy appeared, but is safely moored on the opposite side of the island. The quarters of the Pelican Guards were sunk alongside by a shell day before yesterday. They are now quartered on shore near the battery....

George Nichols Hollins (September 20, 1799-January 18, 1878) became a midshipman in 1814. He served with Commodore Decatur and others, commanded several vessels of his own, and reached the rank of captain September 14, 1855. A sympathizer of Southern causes, he resigned from the U.S. Navy June 6, 1861 and was commissioned as a captain in the Confederate States Navy June 20. By July 31, 1861, he held the rank of commodore and in February 1862 was made flag captain and placed in command of Confederate naval forces operating in the upper Mississippi where he was engaged in the fighting at Columbus, Island No. 10, Fort Pillow, and Memphis. The testimony which follows hereafter is related to those places and instances of engagement. Hollins died in Baltimore of paralysis, recognized as a brave and able officer, a thorough seaman and a worthy gentleman.

Commodore Hollins later reported to a joint special committee of the Confederate Congress investigating the affairs of Confederate Navy Department:

The Tuscarora caught fire going up and was left behind. The Floating Dock had gone up to Island No. 10 and there was blockaded by the enemy. The Red Rover was a boat more for the men to live on board of than for active service. She belonged to the Floating Dock and was merely used for the accommodation of the men to live in. She was not armed at all. If I did not state that the Pontcatrain was there, it was an accidental omission....

Thus, *Red Rover* had been used to house military personnel and not as an armed vessel. As we shall see shortly *Red Rover* would continue her naval career following neither of these usages but a completely different option.

First, however, a bit about the captures made at Island No. 10. In a Confederate list of vessels either destroyed or captured by Federal forces on April 7, 1862, *Red Rover* is identified as a "first class steamboat (old) side-wheel" Such a comment is intriguing in that *Red Rover* was only three years old, the Confederates had paid $30,000 for her, and she was repairable, as previously noted, even from the Confederate perspective.

Equally interesting is the report of *The Scientific American* of April 26, 1862:

We announced in our last number the capture of this somewhat famous island. The full extent of success may be summed up about as follows :

—Prisoners taken; One major-general, two brigadier-generals, seven colonels, eleven lieutenant colonels, fifty-six captains, sixty-four first lieutenants, eighty-one second lieutenants; regimental officers for twelve regiments, about four hundred each; about four thousand sand privates, six hundred and fifty mules, twelve hundred horses, five thousand stand of arms, twenty- four field pieces—six and twelve-pounders, over one hundred pieces heavy artillery, four hundred wagons, and spades, axes, shovels, wheelbarrows, harness, tents and baggage without limit, together with some nine steamboats, valued as follows:

Transport Prince, scuttled $20,000 Transport Ohio Belle, saved $25,000

Transport Red Rover, saved $16,000

Steamer Yazoo, sunk on bar, but will be raised $40,000

Steamer De Soto, saved $60,000 Steamer Mars, saved $46,000

Steamer Admiral, saved $15,000 Steamer Winchester, burned $20,000

Steamer Champion, saved $6,000 Steamer Kanawba Valley, sunk $6,000

John Simmonds, gunboat, sunk $20,000 Grampus, gunboat, sunk $20,000

Mohawk, gunboat, sunk $18,000 Floating Battery, eight guns, saved $30,000

Total $128,000 —Of which there was destroyed $143,000 Total saved $185,000 To which may be added wharf boat and stores… $50,000 Making a grand total of property saved afloat.. $235,000 The capture of this island is one of the most gallant exploits of the war, and reflects great credit upon Commodore Foote, General Pope and all concerned.

In the previous issue, *The Scientific American* had reported:

CAPTURE OF ISLAND NO. 10.

After the evacuation of Columbus by the rebels, they fell back to Island No. 10, which is situated in the Mississippi River, about 45 miles below Columbus, and just south of the line which divides Kentucky from Tennessee. On the Missouri side of the river a few miles below Island No. 10, is the town of New Madrid. The Mississippi is a very crooked stream, and though New Madrid is below Island No. 10, it is nearly in a northwest direction. General Pope marched down the west side of the river and captured New Madrid on the 13th of March, as we have already related. On the 15th of March Commodore Foote came down the river with a fleet of 8 gun-boats and 8 mortar boats, and commenced an attack on the enemy's works. These consisted of 8 batteries mounting 54 guns, and they were aided by a few gunboats and by an immense iron-clad floating battery mounting 16 guns formed of an old floating dock which was constructed at Algiers opposite New Orleans. Commodore Foote commenced a bombardment and cannonade of the rebel batteries which was continued for three weeks, silencing many of the enemy's guns and causing the removal of others. As his gunboats were constructed for fighting with the bow toward the enemy their sterns were not well protected by the iron plates and they were accordingly not well adapted for fighting down stream. The batteries on the island were supported by formidable batteries on the Tennessee shore, and it was soon perceived by Commodore Foote and General Pope that if our army could get in the rear of these batteries and capture them, the place must fall. But the Tennessee shore at this place is a marsh, impassable by an army in the high stage of water which prevailed at that time in the Mississippi, and as the enemy had possession of the river both above and below General Pope, he was unable to procure boats with which to take his army across the river. Our engineers accordingly commenced the survey of the bayous in the vicinity to see if they could find one navigable for steamers of light draft through which boats could be sent to Gen. Pope. These bayous are depressions in the lower valley, or "bottom," as it is called, of the river, and become auxiliary channels or portions of the stream in high water. At the same time Commodore Foote determined upon the desperate enterprise of sending one or more of his gunboats down the stream to run the gauntlet of the enemy's batteries should this measure be necessary. It was found that none of the bayous were navigable, but that one of them, the Chepousi, might be deepened and made navigable by great efforts. This labor was accordingly commenced and the engineers succeeded in getting four steamers and five barges through to New Madrid. In the mean time a violent thunder storm occurred on Sunday evening, April 6, and the gunboat Carondelet, Commander Walke, took the opportunity to make a dash through the enemy's batteries. On the perilous passage 47 shots were fired at her, but fortunately they all missed, and she arrived safely at General Pope's position. With these vessels Gen. Pope crossed the river and marched up stream to the southeast to the rear of the enemy's batteries on the Tennessee shore. About daybreak Monday morning the enemy surrendered, as will be seen by the following official dispatches.

"STEAMER BENTON, OFF ISLAND No. 10, April 7—3:25 A. M. To HON. GIDEON WELLES :—Two officers of the rebel navy have this instant boarded us from Island No. 10, stating, by order of their commanding officer, they were ordered to surrender Island No. 10 to the commander of the naval forces. As these officers knew nothing of the batteries on the Tennessee shore, I have sent Captain Phelps to ascertain something definite on the subject. General Pope is now advancing in strong force to attack the rear. I am ready with the gunboats and mortars to Pt. Ploli in front, Gen. Buford is ready to cooperate; but it seems as if the place is to be surrendered without further defence."

"A.. H. FOOTE, Flag Officer. ST. Louis, Mo., April 8, 1862. To HON. E. M. STANTON, Secretary of War :—General Pope has captured three generals, six thousand prisoners of war, one hundred siege pieces and several field batteries, with immense quantities of small arms, tents, wagons and horses. Our victory is complete and overwhelming. We have not lost a single man. H. W. HALLECK, Major-General."

AS AN ARMY VESSEL

Andrew Hull Foote, the second son of Connecticut Senator Samuel A. and Eudocia Hull Foot, later added "e" to his surname. After a few months at West Point (June-December, 1822), Foote opted for the navy and became an acting midshipman on December 4. A strong call to religion, during a Caribbean cruise in 1827, marked the beginning of the intense reforming spirit of his later years. After cruises in the Mediterranean and around the globe, 1837-41, and two years at the Philadelphia Naval Asylum, he was again in the Mediterranean as first lieutenant of the *Cumberland*. On this vessel he formed a temperance society, did away with the grog tub and made her the first temperance ship in the navy. His example and subsequent exertions were chiefly responsible for abolishment of the spirit ration, finally accomplished in 1862.

In charge of the Brooklyn Navy Yard at the outbreak of the Civil War, Foote had a reputation, not for great brilliance, but for rigid standards of duty and extraordinary persistence. These qualities were tried to the utmost during his command, from August 26, 1861, of naval operations on the upper Mississippi. Though officered by the navy, his flotilla was under army control, and Foote, subject to orders, as he said, "from every brogadoer," overcame incredible difficulties in getting his mortars and twelve gunboats completed, equipped, and manned.

In spite of nervousness and occasional petulance, he had a gentle, lovable nature, and he had also the drive and tenacity essential to successful command.

Federal records indicate the value of the *Red Rover* at time of capture to be $30,000. Commodore Foote (1806-1863), who was born in New Haven, Connecticut, and commanded western flotilla in the Civil War, was in charge of the bombardment, siege, and capture of Island No.10. Foote was given credit for the capture of *Red Rover* and Island No. 10, but it was the Federal Gunboat *Mound City* who took custody of her. On April 9, 1862 Captain A.H.

13

Kilty, Commander of the *U.S.S. Mound City*, wrote to Flag Officer A.H. Foote, Commanding Naval Forces, Western Waters:

> I presume Captain Phelps has informed you of the circumstances under which I took possession of the steamer Red Rover. My engineers and mechanics have been at work on her since yesterday morning, and she will, in a few hours, be in a condition to go to Cairo. One of our shells had passed through all her decks and bottom. Having stopped the leak and pumped her out, she can now, by some repairing, be rendered a serviceable boat. Together with the signal books transmitted to you, I found a mass of papers and letters on board of her, but none of importance. The accompanying package contains the most interesting of the lot. I shall be happy to receive instructions in regard to the disposal of the steamer Red Rover, as I fear, should I leave her, that some of the prowling rebels might burn her....

Under the supervision of Acting Master Cyrenius Dominy, the engineers of the *Mound City* repaired the extensive but not seriously harmful damage that had been inflicted during the Federal bombardment. Once afloat, the *Red Rover* was sent up the Mississippi River to St. Louis where she was fitted out as floating summer hospital for the Western Flotilla.

At the outset of the Civil War medical care was very limited. Although *Red Rover* provided the first support of naval forces as a hospital ship, she was not the first used as a floating hospital during the War of Rebellion. Both the Army and the Sanitary Commission had begun to use steamers and transports as make shift hospitals almost as soon as the war had started. A number of steamers such as the *City of Memphis* were pressed into service as vessels transporting and caring for the sick and wounded. They lacked adequate accommodations and cleanliness as well as sufficient numbers of competent medical personnel. Sanitation and hygiene were so poor, vaccination slow, if available at all, that by the time the war ended in 1865, more men had died from diseases such as malaria, measles, small pox, cholera, typhoid fever, typhus, and dysentery than died of gunshot wounds. Many patients, therefore, could only hope for better facilities when the ship reached port where a hospital might be...an event which might not occur for days or even weeks into the future. Into such chaos sailed the *Red Rover*.

Red Rover's initial service as a hospital ship assigned to the Western Gunboat Flotilla was under the auspices of the Commanding General of the U.S. Army, Lieutenant General Thomas A. Scott who felt that the ships of the Flotilla should work in conjunction with the Army, which was to descend the Mississippi and into the Confederacy. Since such operations were considered to be a part of Army operations and not those of the Navy, the Honorable Gideon Welles, Secretary of the Navy, referred issues regarding the development and building of fleet on the Mississippi and its tributaries—then considered to be western waters—to the War Department. Thus, Commodore John Rodgers, U.S. Navy, via the War Department and Army chain of command, was ordered by Secretary Welles to report to General George B. McClellan to assist in the building of the fleet for the so-called western rivers.

On September 5, 1861, Captain Andrew H. Foote reported to Major General John C. Fremont, U.S. Army as commander of the gunboat flotilla as it then existed…the nucleus of the fleet being the *Tyler*, the *Lexington*, and the *Conestoga*. Foote relieved Rodgers the next day and retained this position until he was disabled by wounds received in the gallant action of Fort Donelson. Foote, who had been appointed by Secretary Welles to be Flag Officer in command of the U.S. Naval Forces, deployed on the Mississippi and the western rivers on November 13, 1861, temporarily turned over his command to Flag Officer Davis on May 9, 1862.

Charles Henry Davis (1807-1877) was born in Boston and appointed a midshipman in 1823. His service included actively directing operations of the Coast Survey along the New England coast. In the Civil War he was fleet captain and chief of staff to S. F. Du Pont in the successful expedition (Nov., 1861) against Port Royal, S.C. As noted above on May 9, 1862, he replaced A. H. Foote in command of the Upper Mississippi flotilla of gunboats. Even though he did not officially assume command until June 17, 1862, on May 10 those under his command repulsed the attack of a Confederate fleet near Fort Pillow, and on June 6 helped annihilate the Confederate fleet before Memphis, taking the city the same day. Later he joined Farragut in an unsuccessful attempt to take Vicksburg. Davis was chief (1862-65) of the Bureau of Navigation and superintendent (1865-67, 1874-77) of the Naval Observatory. For his victories at Fort Pillow and Memphis he was promoted to rear admiral in February 1863.

When *Red Rover* arrived at St. Louis, Army Quartermaster George D. Wise, assigned to the gunboat flotilla, took charge of the fitting out requirements. On May 25, 1862 he wrote to Flag Officer Foote (not knowing he had been replaced by Davis):

My Dear Commodore: Your brother's letter of May 19, with one from General Meigs, which I return, were forwarded to me at this place. I never questioned the propriety of General Meigs requiring of me the usual monthly and quarterly returns and which, however, take an immense amount of labor and a large clerical force. As to the information which he speaks of in his letter to you, I could have any time furnished him with that, and which was sent within three days after being called for. The letter which you so kindly signed for me before leaving Cairo was hurriedly written, principally by Captain Pennock, and was intended to have testified on your part that I had done my duty. Everything is going on very well with me and the quartermaster's department, and I shall soon fill all their requirements. General Meigs has sent me all the money I want. The crews of all the gunboats have been paid off, as well as most of our other indebtedness, and trusting in Providence and your good luck, the gunboat flotilla will arrive to a successful conclusion. I am in St. Louis preparing the Red Rover for a hospital for our sick and wounded. The Sanitary Commission have rendered me valuable advice and aid, and the Red Rover will have every requisite for the purpose [for which] she is intended. I hope to take her in about eight days to Cairo....

The Sanitary Commission to which Wise refers had been established in 1861 to help coordinate the work of voluntary organizations concerned about the health and welfare of military personnel involved in the war. Several pieces of correspondence reflect the relationship between the Sanitary Commission and the fitting out of the *Red Rover*.

The first is a letter from Quartermaster Wise, U.S. Army, to Flag Officer Foote, U.S. Navy, describing the new hospital boat *Red Rover*. From the Office of Naval Depot, Cairo, Illinois he writes on June 10, 1862:

My dear Commodore: ....I wish that you could see our hospital boat, the Red Rover, with all her comforts for the sick and disabled seamen. She is decided to be the most complete thing of the kind that ever floated, and is every way a decided success. The Western Sanitary Association gave us, in cost of articles, $ 3,500. The ice box of the steamer holds 300 tons. She has bathrooms, laundry, elevator for the sick from the lower to the upper deck, amputating room, nine different water-closets, gauze blinds to the windows to keep cinders and smoke from annoying the sick, two separate sick and well, a regular corps of nurses, and two water closets on very deck. We think that the gunboats will have nearly finished their work, and that a different kind will be required for the future. The old boats will be used as floating batteries, to be stationed at New Orleans, Vicksburg, Memphis, and Island No. 10. Fast boats, with light powerful armaments, will act as river police and keep the river open.

Captain Pennock is as busy as usual. Winslow has gone down the river to take command of the Cincinnati. Sanford is now in Cairo, Porter is getting the Essex ready at about twice the expense authorized by you, but if she does not draw too much water will be a very efficient vessel. .....

Alexander Morley Pennock (Oct. 1, 1814-Sept. 20, 1876), born in Norfolk, VA, was left an orphan early in life. Nevertheless, he received a good education and was appointed midshipman from Tennessee on Apr. 1, 1828. Served on *Guerrierre, Natchez, Potomac*, and *Columbia*. Promoted to Lt. in March, 1939 and served aboard the *Decatur, Supply, Marion*, and *Southern Star*. In spite of southern family ties, he remained loyal to the Union and on September 20, 1861 was among senior officers detailed under Capt. A. H. Foote to take over the building of gunboats at St. Louis for the Union Mississippi flotilla. In October, he was made fleet captain in charge of equipment for the flotilla and from early 1862 until the end of 1864, he commanded the naval base at Cairo, IL, where he gained a reputation as one of the best wartime administrative executives of the navy. Admiral C. H. Davis, Foote's successor, wrote, "I cannot use any language too strong to convey a just idea of Capt. Pennock's private and official merit. He is devoted to all his duties, with a simple, honest, straight forward zeal, which gives the performance of them the zest of pleasure." David D. Porter, Davis' relief declared Pennock, "a trump...and worth his weight in gold." Pennock achieved the rank of rear admiral in 1872.

Also on June 10, from the same location, Fleet Captain Alexander M. Pennock reports to Flag Officer Davis regarding the equipment of the hospital boat *Red Rover* as follows:

Sir: The RED ROVER, hospital boat, will leave here tonight or tomorrow. I herewith enclose a list of those employed on board her, which are considered in dispensable necessary. Dr. Bixby, the surgeon, has the highest recommendations, which he will show you, and I would recommend his appointment as surgeon, to date from June 1.

I have given no permanent instructions either to the captain or surgeon, leaving that matter entirely to your superior judgment. I have thanked Captain Wise, assistant quartermaster, for his untiring and successful exertion in the equipment of this boat, and I hope you will approve of all he has done. He informs me that she has stores on board for her crew for three months and medical supplies sufficient for 200 men for three months. She is also abundantly with delicacies for the sick and has on board 300 tons of ice. A barge of ice can be sent down at any time it may be needed.

Captain Wise acknowledges his obligations to the Western Sanitary Commission for the great interest they took in the equipment of this boat, for their advice and substantial aid, to the amount in dollars and cents of $3500 gratuitously bestowed. The boat is supplied with everything necessary for the restoration to health of sick and disabled seamen.

I have directed Captain McDaniel and the surgeon to report to you for orders and for assignment to their particular duties. I think that by mistake I enclosed my letter by the De Soto your letter to me and also that of Mr. Baer, in relations to coal. The quartermaster informs me that no beef could be procured here today to send down by the De Soto.

What instructions shall I give for the future movements of the Bragg and other vessels that may arrive here for repairs?

It should be noted that appointments were sometimes back-dated as Bixby's apparently was. In the above report it is to be noted that Captain Pennock recommended Dr. Bixby on June 12 while in correspondence of June 3 from Bixby to Flag Officer Davis we read:

Dear Sir: Your favor containing my appointment as assistant surgeon in the U.S. gunboat service has been received, and I accept with gratitude this notice you have seen fit to take of me, willing subscribing myself amenable to the laws, regulations, and the dispositions of the Navy as they are or may be established by the Congress of the United States or other competent authority.

In his work, Bixby, who would remain the senior medical officer on *Red Rover* throughout the Civil War, was assisted by fellow Bostonian Dr. George Hopkins and other physicians. Others who are known to have served include:

Michael Bradley
Jacob T. Field
George Lawrence
James S. Knight
William F. McNutt
J. B. Parker
A.W. Pearson
Ninian Pickney
William H. Wilson

Obviously, the ill and wounded had competent doctors to care for them on the *Red Rover* as we shall see as we continue the saga of *Red Rover*'s medical treatment of the troops.

Having noted that the *Red Rover* is now ready for utilization as a hospital ship, on June 14, 1862, Captain Davis, U.S. Navy, issued the following regulations regarding the *Red Rover*:

Hereafter the following regulations will be observed by the vessels of the flotilla in their communications with the hospital boat Red Rover. All sick persons in the fleet are not to be sent on board the hospital boat indiscriminately. It will be understood, on the contrary, that only those patients are to be sent to the hospital boat who it is to be expected to be sick for some time, and those whose cases may require more quiet and better attention and accommodation than can be provided on board vessels to which they belong. Slight disorders and accidents will be treated by the surgeon under whose care they may happen to fall.

This being distinctly understood and uniformly adhered to, following rules will be observed in the transfer of patients to the hospital boat.

1st. When such transfer is necessary in the opinion of the surgeon having care of the case, he will make a brief statement in writing to that effect to the captain of the vessel, who will forward it to the commander in chief. This rule will remain in force as long as there is no fleet surgeon to the flotilla, or as long as the general regulations of the Bureau of Medicine and Surgery cannot be carried into execution.

2d. If the transfer be authorized by the commander in chief, the patient will be accompanied by a statement, giving the name of the vessel to which he belongs, his own name, his rank, the diagnosis and treatment of his disease.

3d. The surgeon having charge of the case will, if possible, go with the patient on board the hospital boat.

4th. The patients on board the hospital boat Red Rover will continue to be borne on the pay and muster rolls of their respective vessels, and will be furnished from their own vessels with whatever they may require in the way of clothing, etc. but their rations will be stopped while on board the hospital boat and credited to the Government.

5th. When restored patients are sent to their proper vessels, they will carry with them a discharge from the hospital boat, signed by the surgeon and attested by the captain of that boat.

Additional. -- Hereafter all applications for ice from the Red Rover must be made between the hours of 8 and 9 o'clock a.m., and no application will be entertained that is made after 9 a.m.

The captain of the Red Rover has been furnished with a list, in accordance with which all supplies of ice will be furnished until further orders.

A letter from Captain Davis to Quartermaster Wise on June 14, 1862, expresses Davis' approval of the new hospital boat Red Rover:

Captain: I have waited until I had an opportunity to make a personal examination of the hospital boat Red Rover before expressing to you my great admiration for your success in this undertaking and the sincere gratitude felt toward you by myself and the other officers and men under my command for the judgment and humanity with which you have executed this important work.

No one but those who have witnessed it can comprehend the sufferings to which are sick have been exposed by the absence of proper accommodation on board the gunboats and by the necessity for frequent and sometimes hasty change of place. The wounded and the patients suffering from fever occupy, under the direction of the surgeon, those parts of the ship which the most quiet and best ventilated. When the ship was cleared for action, as often happened when lying near Fort Pillow, it was necessary to take down their cots and hammocks more than quickly into out-of-way and uncomfortable places. This must always have been attended with pain and distress, if not positive injury. The arrival of Red Rover will put a stop to all of this, promote the efficiency of the squadron by procuring comfort and the means of restoration of the sick. All the conveniences and appliances of the hospital are fully provided, and to these are added the neatness and order essential to so large an establishment. I improve this opportunity to say that I adopt with pleasure your suggestion for creating a coal depot at Memphis, leaving to you the selection of the site for the depot and of the custodian of the coal....

When *Red Rover* reported for duty on June 10, 1862, the stores she had aboard for her crew were sufficient for three months and medical supplies on board were sufficient for two hundred for the same period of time. She was abundantly supplied with special items needed for the caring of the sick. Her icebox carried three hundred tons of ice for her and other ships of the Flotilla to use. While she may seem antiquated or insufficient to us now, *Red Rover* was at the time supplied with everything deemed necessary for the caring of the sick and disabled. It should be noted, also, that in that time hospital ships were not defined nor marked as non-combatants. *Red Rover* was armed with a single thirty-two pounder and was considered ready for any combatant duties that might require her participation. Records show that she served as a guardship and storeship for the fleet, bringing provisions such as fresh meat to the various ships, as well as providing outstanding medical care based on the standards of that day and time.

It was not long before *Red Rover* was actively involved in caring for the sick and the wounded. Her first commanding officer is believed to be a Captain McDaniel but official records provide no further identification of him. There was an Acting Master C. H. Daniels who seems to have fulfilled that role until he resigned in July and Acting Master William R. Welles took command on September 16, 1862. The number of crew members is not consistent. It appears that the ship's complement was twelve officers and thirty-five enlisted. That number stays pretty consistent, although on a given day it would have then, as now, varied perhaps by a person or two. The medical department appears to have varied much more...the usual complement being about thirty but going as high as forty and as low as eight on occasion during her career.

In spite of the disparity in regard to staffing numbers and commanding officers we know that *Red Rover* received her first patient on June 11, 1862— Seaman David Sans, a cholera victim from the Gunboat *Benton*. Four additional patients were take aboard that same day, thirteen more on the twelfth, and thirty-eight more on the thirteenth. *Red Rover* admitted one hundred nine patients June 11-30, and sixty-four of them remained on board the end of June. She admitted two hundred eleven new patients during the July-September quarter and the total patient subsistence amounted to six thousand, two hundred and two days for that period of time. By the end of 1862, *Red Rover* had admitted some three hundred seventy-four patients to her wards. Three hundred twenty-two of them were discharged for further duty, thirty-seven died and five deserted. The total number sick days for patient subsistence was nine thousand eight hundred forty-two. Total expenses for the year were $3462.79.

Red Rover got her first taste of combat conditions on June 17, 1862, when the *Mound City* took part in the successful attack and capture of the Confederate forts at St. Charles, Arkansas, on the White River. The total casualties were one hundred thirty-five out of a total of one hundred seventy-five men on board. A shell from the Confederate batteries, during the action, penetrated the port casement of *Mound City*, killing three men in its flight, and exploded her steam drum. Eight men were scalded to death and forty-tree were either drowned or shot after leaping overboard.. Thirty-seven were transferred to *Red Rover* for transportation to hospitals in Illinois.

Arriving off *Mound City* on the 26th, *Red Rover* put off all but two of the scalded, several other patients and two prisoners of war. One of those transferred ashore was Commander Kilty, commander of the gunboat expedition and of *Mound City* who had been seriously injured by the steam of the exploding boiler.

In his report to Secretary of the Navy Gideon Welles, Flag Officer Davis, writing from the Flagship *Benton* at Memphis on June 20, 1862, provides information regarding the condition of Commander Kilty on board the U.S. hospital boat *Red Rover*:

Sir: The number of wounded men on board the hospital boat Red Rover is 41. The account given me yesterday was incorrect. I shall still wait for further knowledge before presenting a final report of the causalities attending the capture of the St. Charles forts.

The Department will be gratified to learn that the patients are, most of them, doing well. The surgeon assures me that Commander Kilty is out of danger. But he is severely crippled in his hands and feet and suffers a great deal. He is a brave gentleman and a loyal officer. He has always been conspicuous in this squadron for acting his part in the best spirit of the profession. In the attack on the batteries at St. Charles he occupied the leading place and received his wounds at the head of the line in the zealous performance of his whole duty.

Although himself wounded and helpless, he attended the wants and comfort of his injured officers and men. I have gratefully to acknowledge our obligations to Major-General Wallace and to Dr. Robert B. Jessup, of the Twenty-fourth Indiana and to Dr. William

McClellan, of the First Nebraska regiments for their valuable sympathy and assistance.

Sister Angela, the superior of the Sisters of the Holy Cross (some of who are performing their offices of mercy at the Mound City Hospital), has kindly offered the services of the sisters for the hospital boat of this squadron when needed. I have written to Commodore Pennock to make arrangements for their coming. I have the honor to be, very respectively, your most obedient servant.

Based on records of the Order it appears that there were one hundred seventy sisters in the American province of the Order of the Sisters of the Holy Cross. Under Mother Angela Gillespie, eighty of these from twenty-one houses in six States and Washington, D.C., served as nurses in twelve Civil War hospitals, in eight places, there being three hospitals in Memphis and three regimental hospitals with Wallace Brigade in Puducah. Four of the Sisters appear on various muster rolls of the *Red Rover*.

On June 27, 1862, Assistant Surgeon Bixby reported to Davis from the *Red Rover*, then at Mound City:

Dear Sir: In accordance to your order the naval hospital Red Rover left Memphis the 24th instant and arrived at Cairo the 25th. Captain Pennock telegraphed at once to the director of the United States General Hospital at Mound City and procured accommodations for the sick under my charge. In was deemed best for me that night to Mound City to see what accommodations could be found for Captain Kilty. Accordingly, I went, was shown a large room connected with the hospital, but not in the large building. This room is situated on the second story, plenty of light, well ventilated, but not very nice. The next morning I placed the result of my visit before Captain Pennock, who thought it best to look further before deciding.

Yesterday, June 26th, the Red Rover came up to this place, and I put off all but two of the scalded, Mr. Parker, several of my other patients, and two prisoners of war. The day being very warm indeed, I thought best to have Captain Kilty removed as soon as possible; so I accepted the room I saw the night before and saw him safely placed there. I am happy to say, after twelve hours, that he finds himself very comfortable and improving very fast indeed. The men are doing well as could be expected. One has died since the arrival at the hospital.

In my monthly report I will furnish you with the items of our transactions. We hope to be able to return to duty in about six days. Feeling as I ought, I trust, the charge entrusted to me, and a man who has served his country for forty years deserves some little distinction, especially in a helpless situation, I manifested, I must confess, some indecision as to the disposition to be made of Captain Kilty, and I regret to say that such indecision called out some very unpleasant reflections from the medical officer in charge of the hospital, and it not been a case of real necessity, I should have made great efforts to find another place….

Flag Officer Davis wrote three similar messages requesting the dispatching of the *Red Rover* to Cairo. He wrote Commander Pennock:

Sir: The hospital boat Red Rover will report herself at Cairo, and my letters to the captain and surgeon will explain the object of her visit.

To Captain Daniel, the commanding officer of the *Red Rover* he wrote:

Sir: You will proceed tonight with the hospital boat Red Rover to Cairo in tow of the towboats Brown and Shingiss. On your arrival there you will report in person to Commander Pennock, the fleet captain of the squadron, from whom you will receive orders for your further government. Please suggest to him the following changes: First, to put the galley below and open the cabin aft for a circulation of air; second, a steam boiler for the clothes; third, awning for the cabin upper side lights.

Davis also mentioned dispatching the hospital boat *Red Rover* to Cairo were in instructions to Bixby, regarding the disposition of the wounded from the *U.S.S. Mound City*:

> Sir: The hospital boat Red Rover will leave this evening for Cairo. On your arrival there you will report to Commander Pennock and consult with him as to the best method of disposing of the wounded from the gunboat *Mound City*. To transfer them either to the Mound City Hospital or to carry them still farther up to St. Louis seems to me altogether the best plan. Captain Kilty expresses a wish to go to the latter hospital.
>
> Doctor Jones, Pilot Young, Carpenter Manning, and Hospital Steward Seegur will take the earliest boat to Cincinnati, where they will be accompanied by Dr. McNeeley. Captain Wise will furnish them with funds, of which I have given him a memorandum, and for which he will take your receipt.
>
> I leave it to you and Commander Pennock to dispose of any other of the patients in whatever way you think best. It is a source of the deepest gratification to me to know that these poor wounded men are in the hands of so able, attentive, and humane a physician as yourself. I have witnessed your devotion to them with profound gratitude, and I am sure you most enjoy the highest of all rewards, the consciousness of having done your duty....

Lastly, he notified Secretary of the Navy Welles of his action on June 27:

> Sir: It is reported to me this morning that William Cross, seaman, against whom charges were preferred by Lieutenant Commanding Gwin as a spy, has escaped from confinement at St. Louis, Mo. I have the honor to report to the Department that I have sent the hospital boat Red Rover to Cairo, by advice of the medical officers of the fleet. The scalded patients suffered excessively from the heat of the weather....

Bixby replied to Davis' comments regarding the wounded from the *U.S.S. Mound City* in a letter dated June 27:

> Dear Sir: I can not resist acknowledging, with the deepest gratitude, your kind approbation of my humble efforts toward the unfortunate victims of the past week. While your words send. a thrill of encouragement. through the heart of one anxious to serve his country, yet he feels that in the performance of one's plain and positive duty there lies no merit. The satisfaction of having endeavored to do duty is mine, which, as you truly remark, is the greatest reward. our time, I am Trusting I may be pardoned for this trespass on your time....

In the meantime Commander Pennock, Navy, wrote Davis on June 26 regarding affairs at Cairo:

> Sir: ....The sternpost of the Red Rover is broken from the keel up, and she will have to be hauled out on the ways for repairs. I hope to have the Sumter ready to leave bySunday. We shall then be able to increase the force on the Bragg and have her ready in a short time....

In his June 20 letter above, Davis mentioned to Welles Sister Angela and the Sisters of the Holy Cross. It appears that the medical assistance provided by these angels of mercy was done at the shore hospitals initially. To care for the wounded on the up-river trip and assist in their transfer to hospitals ashore, Doctor Bixby was able to obtain approval of his request for male nurses from the Army Mortar Fleet then stationed at Memphis. It was also about this time that Sister Angela, the Superior of the Sisters of the Holy Cross, offered the services of the Sisters for the hospital boat. Flag Officer Davis wrote to Fleet Officer Pennock asking that arrangements for their coming might be made. It is clear that Sisters of the Holy Cross were on board the *Red Rover* during her service in the summer of 1862. Their letters published in Sister M. Eleanore's *On the King's Highway* (New York, 1931) show that Sister M. Anthanasius served six weeks prior to October, 1862, and others were "on board for awhile." There is, however, no conclusive evidence that women were regularly attached as nurses in the Medical Department of the *Red Rover* prior to the time that she was fitted out and commissioned as a hospital ship at the end of 1862. More will be said later about these wonderful angels of mercy who were, in reality, the forerunners of the Navy Nurse Corps.

Red Rover completed repair of the broken sternpost by July 8 and left Mound City to join the rest of the Western Flotilla, then above Vicksburg. She arrived there July 12.

Early on July 12, the ships of the Western Flotilla moved into the Yazoo River, heading upstream. The gunboats were preparing for action, when at about 6 a.m., they discovered the powerful Confederate ironclad ram *Arkansas* coming toward them from the opposite direction. The Confederate ship successfully passed through the entire Federal Western Flotilla and the Ram Fleet, leaving many, many causalities in her wake. Numbers of these men were treated aboard *Red Rover*, which remained in the area while the Union forces engaged the Confederates at Vicksburg.

The battle for Vicksburg was of significance to both sides and is recorded in various annals of the conflict. Here we would report some of the official correspondence.

First there is the report of Captain H. Walke U.S. Navy, commanding *U.S.S. Carondelet*, transmitting the abstract log of the gunboat for July 22, 1862. From *Mound City*, on September 4, he writes:

> Sir: I herewith enclose a copy of the remarks in the log book of this vessel on the morning of July 22, 1862. Mr. Brennand, the first master of this vessel, and Mr.Deming,the pilot, were on the point opposite Vicksburg when the Essex passed the Arkansas. I was on the Red Rover and saw our fleet engage the enemy and the Essex pass out of gunshot below the rebel batteries some time before the firing between our fleet and the enemy had ceased. The ways here are still occupied by the prize General Price, with most of the mechanics and laborers cutting off her upper works. The tugs are being hauled out and repaired on the remaining ways. The Carondelet is being repaired as fast as possible, but she will be detained longer than was expected, I fear. A large number of our

officers and crew are still sick. I beg leave to be considered an applicant for the ram Fort Henry or Choctaw, now being built at St.. Louis.

Two excerpts from the log are provided. From the entry of July 15, we learn that "…four men were killed, 15 wounded, and 16 missing. Expended 90 rifle and solid shots. From 8 to 12 meridian: Came to anchor with fleet. At 8:30 hospital boat Red Rover came off alongside and took off the wounded."

The July 22 entry does not specially mention the *Red Rover* but relates data regarding the conflict:

July 22, 1862.—From 4 to 8 a. in.: At 4, Benton, Louisville, Cincinnati, and GeneralBragg lying off the point above Vicksburg. At 4:15 Essex got underway and started down the river. 4:20, rams Queen of the West and Switzerland underway, the Queen going down the river. 4:30, fleet opened fire upon the rebel fortifications, Essex passing below the point. At 5, ram Queen of the West returning up the river. 5:15, in ceased on both sides. 5:30, fleet returning up the river; Louisville came alongside of coal barge astern of us. Benton, Cincinnati, and General Bragg coming to an anchor in shoal water on the other bank of the river. Essex passed the batteries, and seen lying below the rebel batteries. T. S. GILLMORE, Fourth Master.

An abstract of the log of the *U.S.S. Benton* records a near tragedy on *Red Rover* on August 29: "At 5 p. m. the hospital boat Red Rover was seen to be on fire. Sent away all the boats and assisted in putting it out."

The cause and severity of the fire are not known, but *Red Rover* seems to have been disabled only temporarily. While the fire was certainly disruptive, it appears to have caused inconvenience more than anything serious.

On September 16, Commodore Davis, while aboard the Flagship *Eastport*, then at Helena, Arkansas, wrote Wm. R. Wells, appointing him first master in gunboat service:

Sir: Enclosed you will find your appointment as first master in the gunboat service. If you accept the same, you will report to me immediately for duty aboard the hospital boat Red Rover., now lying off Helelna, and will execute the enclosed oath, which when taken and signed, will be forwarded to me to be forwarded to Washington for the files of the Department, in compliance with the terms of the law.

Wells, from Burlington, Iowa, accepted the appointment and as the Acting Master was ordered to take command of *Red Rover*, then laying off Helena, Arkansas. He would later be promoted to Acting Volunteer Lieutenant so he obviously was capable of doing what was asked of him by his superiors.

On September 18, Commodore Davis, in connection with the proposed fitting of the U.S. ship *Red Rover* for the winter, ordered Fleet Captain Pennock as follows:

Sir: This letter will be handed you by Dr. Bixby, of the Red Rover, who will present you at the same time with a paper containing his views upon the changes necessary to adapt the hospital boat to the coming season. These views in general meet my approval. I think you had better, for special reasons connected with the Sanitary Commission, have the Red Rover go to St. Louis for repairs. My approval of Dr. Bixby's views will not prevent you from making any alteration you make think necessary.

The same day Commodore Davis sent a letter to James E. Yeatman, President of the Western Sanitary Commission, headquartered at St. Louis, acknowledging the Commission's kindness and attention to the sick on the hospital ship:

Sir: The present season is about drawing to a close, and upon the recommendation of Dr. Bixby, I have sent the hospital boat Red Rover to St. Louis to be properly fitted up for the winter.

I cannot let her return to your vicinity without expressing, in behalf of myself and the officers of the vessels under my command, our heartfelt and grateful acknowledgments of your uniform kindness and attention to the wants and comforts of the sick of this squadron.

I beg you to make known to the Sanitary Commission, of which you are president, that we are all deeply sensible of the uniform and unremitting watchfulness and care which you have extended toward us. Your contributions have not only materially contributed to the comforts, the needs, and the essential improvement of the sick, but they have done a great deal toward relieving the irksomeness of confinement, by delicacies suited to the fastidious appetites of the sick and by supplying them both occupation and amusement. I beg you to believe that your benevolent labors in our behalf have been fully appreciated.

The next day Commodore Davis sent word to First Master A.M. Grant, commanding the *New National*, ordering the transportation of fragments of guns to be presented to the Sisters of the Holy Cross.

Sir: I wish you to stop at Island No. 10 and take on board the fragments of a gun known as Lady Davis, which burst in the hands of the rebels. I wish you to stop again at Columbus and to take on board the fragments of a gun known as the Lady Polk, which also burst in the hands of the rebels; the fragments of this gun are lying on the bank near Mr. Davis's house. You will exhibit the enclosed letter from General Quinby to myself to the military commanders at Island No. 10 and Columbus, who will have the goodness to allow you to take away the fragments above designated. Please explain to them that they are to be placed at the disposal of Sister Angela, superior of the Sisters of the Holy Cross, who are the principal nurses in our military hospitals and that they are to be recast into a statue of peace for one of the religious establishments of which Sister Angela is the superior. You will carry these fragments of guns to Cairo and deliver them to the care of Captain Pennock.

On Christmas Eve, 1862, Sister M. Veronica (C. Moran), Sister M. Adela (M. Reilly), and Sister M. Callista (E. Pointan) transferred to *Red Rover* from the Army Hospital at Mound City. It is believed that Sisters Veronica and Adela tended the sick on the hospital ship until November 15, 1865, the last day of service for the *Red Rover*, which provided medical care for only three less than 2500 patients during the war. Sister M. John (C. McLouglin) carried on reports as Sister St. John joined the others on February 9, 1863, and served as a nurse on the *Red Rover* until September 30, 1863. For unknown reasons Sister M. Callista left the hospital ship on March 2, 1863, but reported on board for duty again on January 28, 1865. At least two female Negro nurses worked under the direction of the Sisters on board the *Red Rover* when she was commissioned. They were Alice Kennedy and Sarah Kinno. Those serving later were Ellen Campbell, Betsy Young, and Dennis Downs. These women may truly be said to be the pioneers or forerunners of the United States Navy Nurse Corps as they were the first female nurses carried on board a United States Navy Hospital Ship. In addition to the valiant nurses there were several laundresses employed in the Hospital Department of the ship. Referred to in official records as "sundry employees hired by the Medical Department" they were not always mustered since they "cannot strictly be said to belong to the service." Nonetheless, they were carried on some muster rolls as well as on invoices under the heading of "Amounts paid persons 'not shipped' on board U.S.N. Hospital Red Rover employed in the Medical Department." Their number, including men employed, varied, as noted earlier, from the peak of approximately forty in the busiest times to as few as eight. Muster rolls of the *Red Rover* show that nurses—male and female alike—sister and lay were paid fifty cents a day while Army nurses were only paid forty cents daily. Shortly after the war, on June 9, 1865, Fleet Surgeon Pinkney wrote to the chief nurse at Pinkney Hospital:

Dear Sister St. John: Will you do me the favor to forward to Mother Angela with the best regards of Fleet Surgeon Pinkney the enclosed emblem (a gold cross) as evidence of his high appreciation of one who has the honor to represent as its head the noblest of the good ones of the earth.

As time went by, it was discovered that the work of the Flotilla was more naval than land. The officers were naval, most of the men sailors, and much of the ordnance and other stores supplied the Navy Department. There appears to have been no severe or harmful disharmony in spite of the fact that at times there was confusion and embarrassment due to inter-service nature being utilized. Congress, on July 16, passed an act which transferred the Western Gunboat Flotilla to the Navy Department. Secretary of the Navy Welles notified Commodore Davis on September 10 that October 1 would be the day the official transfer of the Western Flotilla from the War to the Navy Department would occur, a move agreed to by the War Department.

At the same time, the name of the Flotilla was changed to that of the Mississippi Squadron. Acting Rear Admiral David D. Porter was appointed Commander of the Squadron, effective the date of transfer, but he did in reality take command until October 15. The ships that were transferred to the Navy included ten iron-clad gunboats, eight wooden gunboats, eight transport steamers, including *Red Rover*, thirteen steam tugs, two ammunition steamers, and one large barge type boat of four thousand tons used as a wharf at the Naval Depot, Cairo. Thus, on October 1, 1862, the United States Navy acquired its first hospital ship, the *U.S.S. Red Rover*.

While all this administrative process was taking place, an Illinois Prize Court, which had jurisdiction over the *Red Rover* as a prize of war, sold her, on September 20, to the Navy Department for the sum of $9,314.28. Such was a bargain price considering she had been valued at $30,000 when purchased by the Confederacy in 1861 and captured by the Union at Island No. 10.

Red Rover arrived at the Naval Depot, Cairo on September 23 to be fitted for winter use. On September 26, she transferred to the Army Hospital, Mound City, eighty patients, half of whom were ravaged by disease and fever and unfit for service. Correspondence regarding the availability of adequate medical facilities is indicative of the conditions at the time.

Dr. Edward Gilcrist, Fleet Surgeon, provides, on September 24, the following picture:

> Sir: I have the honor to enclose a copy of a letter from Doctor Franklin, the surgeon at Mound City Hospital, from which you will perceive that no more of our sick can be received there. It is absolutely necessary that the sick of the Red Rover hospital boat be removed before any repairs or alterations be commenced on board

the vessel. I do not think that our sick now in the hospital at Mound City and Cairo can much longer be accommodated there. For these reasons, and considering the large number of sick now destitute of proper accommodations, and taking into account also the probable necessities of the service for some time to come, I respectively recommend that the building mentioned to Doctor Franklin be procured and immediately established as a naval hospital....

(subenclosure)

U.S. General Hospital.
Mound City, Ill., September 24, 1862

Sir: I have the honor to inform you that we have at present no hospital facilities for the 130 seamen you propose sending here; all our beds are filled excepting about one dozen. The Mound City Hotel, a building capable of holding some 250 patients, can be taken possession of by competent authority, which can be a good building for hospital purposes. I should think the building could be hired at nothing over $1,500 per year, as it has paid its proprietors scarcely nothing for the investment. The foundry, a brick building capable of holding 400 patients, can also be taken possession of by Government authorities, if they deem it practical. Either of these buildings will make good hospitals, the former with but a little outlay of money; the latter will require a considerable sum to put it in order for a hospital, which will deprive the Government of its use for some weeks. The hotel can be occupied in forty-eight hours after getting possession. I leave the consideration of these two buildings to the naval depot, and remain, Very respectfully, your obedient servant, E. C. Franklin, Surgeon U.S. Army.

Months before, Commodore Foote had taken the initial step toward organizing a Navy Medical Department. From the gunboat *Essex*, on January 2, 1862, he wrote to Secretary Welles:

> Sir: I respectively request that Surgeon Andrew A. Henderson may be ordered to this Flotilla as Fleet Surgeon. In view of the service in which the Flotilla is engaged, and there being no Naval Surgeon attached to it, I consider the appointment of a Fleet Surgeon desirable alike on the ground of securing good medical treatment and surgery and a judicious and economical expenditure of medical stores.

Gilcrist in consultations with Army Surgeon Franklin at the Mound City Hospital and the Medical Director of the District became convinced that co-operative arrangements for the caring of the Squadron's sick was absolutely necessary. He reported to Dr. William Whelan, Chief of the Bureau of Medicine and Surgery:

> Heretofore, from the nature of the case there has been ever conceivable irregularity in the medical affairs of the squadron and the service would have suffered excessively but for the cheerful and zealous assistance which the medical officers of the Army have always been ready to give us, frequently to their own great inconvenience. The plan proposed will not only relieve them of a great amount of duty and responsibility which properly belongs to us, but is the only one, I am convinced, for the sole organization and management of the medical duty of the Squadron as to deserve your approbation.

Gilchrist assured Whelan that the Army would continue to furnish medical stores for the Squadron as in the past. He further reassured Whelan that the proposal was entirely approved by both Fleet Captain Pennock and Rear Admiral Davis.

Administrative action came forth quickly. On September 29,1862, Davis requested authorization from the Bureau of Medicine and Surgery for the delivery of the building for a Naval Hospital, informing him that the "senior medical officer of the Army says our sick numbering 300 must be moved from the Mound City Hospital." In a few days approval was granted and the Mound City Hotel was rented for $75 per month. This marked the beginning of the organization for the Navy Medical Department on western waters. Even though Davis had on June 14, 1862 (see above), issued regulations for the *Red Rover*, few, if any, instructions had been issued to the Service for the regulation of medical departments which was "half Navy and half Army." Irregularities and confusion resulted more from lack of direction and written instructions for carrying out uniform procedures than from ignorance or unawareness of regulations. When the transfer of the Western Flotilla from Army to Navy took place, many surgeons of the Medical Service of the Navy were caught up in the irregularities brought about by this lack of uniformity. Davis immediately resolved the problem by requesting that Regulations of the Service be sent for use throughout the Squadron. He further requested the forms used by the Bureau of Medicine and Surgery so that all surgeons and medical personnel of the Mississippi Squadron could better and more efficiently serve the Navy.

On October 23 Gilchrist wrote to Dr. Whelan:

The fitting up of the Hospital and Hospital Boat; the care of a great number of sick for whom I had no proper accommodation and the labor of surveying all the sick of the Squadron in this vicinity has brought upon me an amount of work, which has made it impossible hitherto, for one to make such regular and accurate reports to you as I could otherwise have done. Some time must still elapse before the Hospital Department of the Squadron can be regularly and properly organized. It involves a greater amount of labor than anyone not upon the spot can readily comprehend.

On November 12, Gilcrist again wrote to Dr. Whelan:

All the sick in this vicinity, belonging to the Squadron have been surveyed.... The Naval Hospital at Mound City and the Hospital Boat at that place are now full to overflowing, and the Ordnance Boat *Judge Torrence* is now being converted into a hospital boat for temporary service.

From a report of Captain Pennock, dated Dec 23, 1862, from Cairo, Ill, we learn:

...The New Era will be sent down to-morrow evening. The Red Rover will join you by the 30th instant. The Judge Torrence will leave to-morrow evening.... I have made the following changes in the disposition of officers: I have ordered Acting Assistant Surgeon Vail to the New Era. I have ordered Acting Master's Mate H. G. Warren (formerly purser's steward of the Little Rebel) to the New Era. William Wharry, acting master's mate, ordered by you to report to me for duty on the U.S. gunboat Glide, I have ordered to the New Era, there being great want of officers for that boat.

In December Ninian Pickney became the Fleet Surgeon, relieving Edward Gilcrist. Pinkney would continue Gilcrist's excellent work. Also in December, on the 26, *Red Rover* was officially commissioned as the first U.S. Navy Hospital Boat. It was not long until she returned to the heat of battle.

In the meantime Davis had been succeeded, officially on Oct. 15, 1862, by Admiral David Dixon Porter (1813-1891). Porter had served under his father, David, in the Mexican War before he was appointed in 1829 as a midshipman in the U.S. Navy. He held his first command, the *Spitfire*, during the Mexican War. In the Civil War he led the mortar flotilla of the Union fleet commanded by David Farragut in the successful assault on New Orleans in 1862. He contributed to Ulysses S. Grant's success in the Vicksburg campaign in 1863. For these services on the Mississippi River he was made rear admiral. He cooperated (1864) with Gen. Nathaniel P. Banks in the Red River. Next to Farragut, Porter was deemed by some to be the most outstanding Union naval commander. As superintendent (1865-69) of the U.S. Naval Academy he proved himself an able organizer and administrator. Porter was promoted to vice admiral in 1866; in 1870, on Farragut's death, he became full admiral.

Equally distinguished and involved was Gideon Welles (1802-1878). Born in Glastonbury, Connecticut, he was editor and part owner of the *Hartford Times*, one of the first New England papers to support Andrew Jackson. One of the organizers of the Jacksonian forces in Connecticut, Welles served in the state legislature, was three times elected state comptroller of public accounts and was postmaster of Hartford. He also served as chief of the Bureau of Provisions and Clothing for the U.S. Navy (1846-49). Welles left the Democratic party over the slavery issue, helped found (1856) the *Hartford Evening Press*, a Republican paper, and in 1861 became Secretary of the Navy in Abraham Lincoln's cabinet. Honest, sincere, and fearless, Welles was never just a time server. He was also shy, averse to close association with his fellow human beings. He was severely critical of their faults, detecting their faults instead of looking for virtues. He had a gift of insight in his ability to appraise men. As one who was incorruptible, efficient, and something of a curmudgeon, Welles built the powerful Union navy of the Civil War. The construction of the *Monitor* and the other ironclads resulted largely from his support, and the victorious admirals David C. Farragut and David D. Porter were men of his choice. Welles was one of the first to recognize Lincoln's essential greatness, he thoroughly disliked some of his cabinet colleagues, notably William H. Seward and Edwin M. Stanton. He was a moderate who favored Lincoln's Reconstruction plan and, retaining his post under Andrew Johnson, stood by the new President in his struggle with the radical Republicans in Congress even though he did eventually return to the Democratic Party.

AS A NAVY SHIP

In December, 1862, Fleet Surgeon Ninian A. Pinkney relieved Fleet Surgeon Edward Gilchrist. Pinkney made the *Red Rover* his headquarters ship and from her flowed the orders, correspondence, pleas, and action of this remarkable man as he overcame the difficulties and problems obstructing the proper care of the sick and wounded of the Mississippi Squadron. To the Chief of the Bureau of Medicine and Surgery went recommendations for organization and standard instructions to surgeons of the squadron. Acting in concert with Admiral Porter and Fleet Officer Pennock, he emphasized the need of supplying all the ironclads with medical officers and the light-draft ships with surgeon stewards so that these fighting ships on frequent detached duty could properly care for their sick and wounded until they reached the *Red Rover* or shore hospitals. No opportunity of improving the service seemed to escape Pinkney's attention. Typical is a letter written aboard the *Red Rover* on February 7 which reads in part:

> The fourth paragraph of the Section seventeenth of Regulations, if literally construed and applied to this Hospital Ship, absolutely requires that patients having injury or disability likely to entitle them to pensions, or determined by survey, must remain in the hospital until their claim for pension shall have been forwarded to the Department, acted upon, and the decision officially made known to the Fleet Surgeon by it. I desire to be instructed whether such instruction is imperative timely binding for the reason that if applied to this Squadron it must give rise to exposure to an unhealthy climate (which might be avoided), liability to overcrowding of the Hospital and overworking of attendants, and serving unnecessary accumulation of accounts here all of which are serious evils.

Seven months later he had lost none of his zeal or concern for men of the squadron when he wrote Dr. Whelan, the Chief of Bureau of Medicine and Surgery:

> I have the honor to acknowledge receipt of your communication directing the appointment of competent Surgeon Stewards to the charge of the Medical Department of such vessels where the Medical Officers could be dispensed with. I shall in accordance with this order carry out its provisions as far as may be found practicable. I do not think, however, that any reduction can safely be made in the Medical Department of this Squadron, as all of the vessels are placed on separate service.
>
> From the nature of the climate, it is reasonable to suppose that Medical Officers are equally liable to attacks of sickness as other officers; and therefore would require leave of absence. There are at present several whose state of health is such as to require change of climate. Their services cannot well be dispensed with until I can obtain medical officers to take their place.
>
> The increased compensation to Surgeon Stewards will enable me to obtain the services of competent men, who can safely take charge of the Medical Department of the smaller vessels.

Ninian Pinkney (June 7, 1811-December 15, 1877) was born in Annapolis, MD, where his father was involved in local politics. Pinkney graduated from St. John's College in Annapolis in 1830 and from Jefferson Medical College, Philadelphia, as an MD in 1833. It was expected that Pinkney would stay on and teach at Jefferson but he chose instead to join the navy where he was commissioned as assistant surgeon in 1834. He served until 1840 when he was court-martialed on charges of "disrespectful and provoking language to a superior" and "conduct unbecoming to an officer and gentleman." Found guilty he was suspended for eight months but returned to duty thereafter, serving faithfully. Pinkney was assigned in 1862 to Admiral Porter's Mississippi Squadron as surgeon of the fleet. As such there were over eighty ships were under his supervision. In a letter to his wife, he mentions traveling some 8,000 miles in the process of carrying out his duties. That Pinkney Hospital in Memphis was so named by Admiral Porter in his honor attests to his ability.

While *Red Rover* watched over the sick and wounded above Vicksburg in the winter of 1862-63, additional disabled accumulated along the rivers without means of providing for them. Memphis was the most central point, as well as the most healthy place on the Mississippi River, so permission was requested for the Navy to occupy any suitable buildings at Memphis for hospital purposes.

General Grant promptly ordered that a former Confederate building be turned over to Fleet Surgeon Pinkney. All hospital buildings, save for the Mound City Hotel, were in the possession of the Army, and those being full to overflowing, there was little possibility of accommodating the Navy sick without scattering them all over the country, removing some at the risk of their lives.

Thus, the Commercial Hotel of Memphis was converted to hospital use by the Navy. The hotel was soon providing shelter to 248 men. It was named Hospital Pinkney in honor of the fleet surgeon. Sister St. John left the *Red Rover* at the end of September to take charge of the nursing there. Hotel Pickney answered the earlier plea of Fleet Surgeon Gilcrist that the sick of the Mississippi Squadron be brought together at a place where they could receive care of the exclusive direction of naval medical officers.

In the meantime, *Red Rover* had gotten under way on December 29, heading downstream. She arrived at Memphis and reported to Captain Bishop, General Officer of the Port, whose office was aboard the General Bragg. *Red Rover* received five crew members from the General Bragg and the paymaster approved the purchase of some fresh meat to be used on board. The price of eight cents a pound provides an interesting side note.

Continuing downstream, *Red Rover* joined the expedition up the White River. While Federal forces were taking the Port of Arkansas (Fort Hindman), she stayed at the mouth of the River to receive the wounded. During her departure, she was fired upon by the Confederates and two shots found their way into the hospital area of the ship but there were no casualties.

Official records of this period include General Order No. 30, of January 7, 1863. Acting Rear Admiral David D. Porter instructed the White River forces as follows:

> In ascending the White and Arkansas rivers the following order
> will be observed: Lieutenant-Commander Watson Smith will go

ahead in the Rattler, sounding with two leads, and when he comes to shoal water (less than 9 feet) he will hoist the cornet. If he can [sic] through with that depth of water he will hoist the blue jack. The Romeo, the Juliet, and Forest Rose will follow the Rattler, sounding with two leads, their guns trained forward of the [sic] and the fuzes cut to one second. The Marmora will go ahead of this ship, sounding, and the guns similarly prepared. Vessels will not wait for orders to fire when they see the enemy's troops or when fired upon. Commanders will look out for torpedoes or floats or wires extending from the bank. Boats will be kept manned to remove them. The Louisville, Baron De Kalb, and Cincinnati will come after this vessel. The Signal will cover the twentieth transport and the Lexington will bring up the rear. The *Red Rover* and Torrence will remain at the mouth of White River and guard it and the coal barges, notifying any light-draft gunboats and all coal or store boats to stop at the mouth of White River until further orders. The cornet over the jack will signify danger near from the enemy.

Acting Rear-Admiral Porter, in Report No. 57, Navy, provided Gideon Welles information regarding the disposition of the vessels of his command, that is, the U.S. MISSISSIPPI SQUADRON, on the Arkansas River as of January 16, 1863:

SIR: The following is the disposition of the squadron at the present time: The Black Hawk, Louisville, Chillicothe, Rattler, Glide, and Linden are off Fort Hindman, Arkansas River. The Baron DeKalb, Cincinnati, Signal, Romeo, and Forest Rose are up White River, at St. Charles, which place they have taken possession of. The Marmora and Juliet have just returned from the mouth of the Yazoo, where they were sent to convoy coal. The Carondelet is at Island No. 10, where the New Era has gone to relieve her. The Judge Torrence and Great Western, powder vessels, and the Sovereign, store vessel, and the Red Rover, hospital ship, are at the mouth of this river....

On January 24, 1863 writing from the mouth of the Yazoo River, Admiral Porter admonishes Acting Master Wells, commanding U.S. hospital ship *Red Rover*, regarding the showing of lights contrary to general orders:

> SIR: Your attention is called to General Order No. 4, in relation to showing lights. At 11 o'clock at night your ship was showing lights in every officer's room and in every office, and your ship a fair target for anyone to shoot at. No lights will be allowed in the Texas after 8 o'clock at night, and not then if the officers do not screen them. I look to you to see that no lights are shown in your vessel except those that are absolutely necessary. Have no lights moving about decks, and hang, also, canvas around and in front of your boilers, if you have it.

Red Rover continued to support the Fleet—caring for the sick and wounded of the ships of the Squadron from February to the fall of Vicksburg in July 1863. She was also a provisions ship in that she was able to provide fresh meat and ice to the other ships as she moved from place to place. She also sent medical personnel ashore when and wherever needed as providing personnel for burial details.

On April 16 *Red Rover* weighed anchor and proceeded down the Mississippi, landing on the Louisiana shore just above Vicksburg at 10:15 p.m. The Squadron gunboats and transports passed her with the intention of running the blockade past Vicksburg. They rounded the point about 11 p.m. and enemy musketry opened up. Then the Confederates' heavy guns roared out as fires were lighted on shore to illuminate the passing Squadron. The gunboats bombarded the Vicksburg batteries as they swept ahead at full speed and succeeded in breaking through the blockade.

Moving from the scene of combat, the *Red Rover*, filled to capacity with patients, steamed to Memphis, arriving on April 23. Here she transferred her most serious cases to Hospital Pinkney and prepared to make repairs in the Navy Yard. On May 20, with her repairs completed and eleven men from Hospital Pinkney added to her crew, the hospital ship again set out for Vicksburg. She arrived off the White River the next morning and Fleet Surgeon Pinkney came aboard to accompany her to the mouth of the Yazoo. She continued to receive, treat and evacuate the wounded of the fleet as the campaign against the Confederates continued into July. Vicksburg fell on July 4. Ten days later the *Red Rover* arrived at Memphis with the casualties of the successful siege. By the end of July she was again anchored at Vicksburg. On July 31 she proceeded down river to the Jefferson Davis Plantation and transferred medicine to the gunboat *Carondelet*, thence to Grand Gulf, Mississippi, where she delivered medical supplies to the gunboat *Louisville*. Continuing down river she visited Natchez, Baton Rouge and New Orleans, then proceeded back up river by way of the various fleet rendezvous to Memphis where she tied to shore near the Navy Yard on August 15,1863.

Again in need of repairs, the *Red Rover* remained at Memphis until October 17. On the 19th she came to anchor off Mound City, and officers came on board to hold a survey of the hospital ship and her machinery. Only three patients were on board as of the first of the month and only 21 patients were admitted to her care for the remainder of the year while the ice ran heavy in the river and she waited for extensive repairs. She did not get on the ways of the shipyard until February 23, 1864, and came off on March 10. She left the yard on April 11, shifting to Cairo where her commanding officer, Acting Volunteer Lieutenant William R. Wells, reported to Fleet Captain Pennock. Here the *Red Rover* received medical stores for the fleet and the sick men from the steamer *Clara Dolson*. She stood down river on April 12 as the Federal troops at Fort Pillow, Tennessee, were overwhelmed by the Confederates. An agreement was reached to allow the Union Army to remove their wounded and bury their dead on the morning of April 13. About fifty of the wounded were placed on board the *Platte Valley*. Those who could walk were brought down the bluffs, supported on either side by a Confederate soldier. Other Union prisoners were sent in from Confederate camps after the *Platte Valley* departed.

The *Red Rover* landed at Fort Pillow at 2 p.m., taking aboard all the wounded (13 soldiers) for care in hospital wards. She readied her gun for action and prepared for an expected attack from the guns of Fort Randolph as she headed back up river, but she passed that Confederate fort without incident. She arrived at Memphis on the morning of April 14, sending the wounded soldiers to the Army Hospital and the sick seamen of the Squadron to Hospital Pinkney. She started back down river the next day, putting off medical stores and supplies to ships of the squadron at such places as the mouth of the White and Yazoo Rivers and the Jefferson Davis Plantation below Vicksburg.

On April 17 the *Red Rover* anchored at the mouth of Red River to support the fleet cooperating with the Army in the expedition up that stream. Leaving the *Red Rover* at anchor, the fleet gunboats headed up the river. Upon reaching Springfield, Louisiana, they found that Union land forces were falling back towards Grand Ecore. The gunboats were obliged to return down river as they had no infantry to dislodge the Confederate batteries that could be mounted on the river banks. On the return voyage they were frequently fired upon by the Confederates from every assailable point. Upon reaching Grand Ecore the gunboats found that the Red River had fallen so low that they could not pass over the rapids. It seemed that the better part of the squadron would he doomed to destruction as the Union Army prepared to evacuate that place. Lieutenant Colonel Joseph Bailey, Acting Engineer of the Nineteenth Army Corps, proposed a plan for building a series of dams across the rocks of the falls, thus raising the level of the river. Constructed by Army and Navy men, the dam had a center opening which let the ships ride out on the crest of the water. On May 9 the gunboat *Lexington* passed into calm water, soon followed by the rest of the fleet. Meantime the *Red Rover*, stationed at the mouth of the Red River, delivered medical supplies, ice provisions and stores to ships of the fleet as she admitted their sick and wounded to her hospital department.

In late June, Rear-Admiral Porter provided the following guidance to those under his command:

> The enemy are about to evacuate Vicksburg in front in boats, while a force of 12,000 rebels attempt to take possession of the point opposite the city and Joe Johnston attacks the rear of the army at Vicksburg. The gunboats and Switzerland will move up to the canal, ready at night to steam up, and if the enemy attempt to cross over, push in amongst the boats and destroy them and all in them; there will be no time to pick any one up. The lower gunboats will confine their fire to the river and the banks on the Vicksburg side, for fear of injuring our troops, who will be down at the point in force. In case our troops are driven back, they will fall back on the levee, where the 30-pounder battery was; and if, at night, will send up rockets, when our lower vessels will open fire on the roads and to the left of the woods, but to the right of the levee. Tar barrels will be prepared by the vessels to light up the levee from the houses

where the mortars were last year to a little below the canal. A perfect understanding must be had with the officers of the Marine Brigade, that the commanders may know their exact position in the woods. The Rattler will remain at Milliken's Bend and be prepared to cover our troops there, the captain going on shore and making himself acquainted with the localities. He will place what vessels I send up there to enfilade the enemy as he approaches and attacks. The Argosy will hold herself in readiness to go to Milliken's Bend or other place, as she may be wanted. The Mamiton will drop down abreast of the Black Hawk, lying near the Louisiana side, with all her port guns run out and one bow gun. The Lexington and Choctaw will be ready to drop down at a moment's notice where the mortar boats are, and be prepared to fire in the direction of Vicksburg to cut up the enemy as he comes across the land, or to take position above the canal to cut off the rebels that may come from Richmond, [La.]. The Great Western will haul out in the stream at her usual place and be prepared to fire shells over the tents 900 yards to the rear. The *Red Rover* will take position a little above Young's Point, and be prepared to fire shells 1,400 yards to the rear of that point. Lieutenant-Commander Breese will see that crews are provided from the different vessels for the two scows with guns, and will have a tug along-side of each one at night ready to drop them out in the middle of the stream or near the side we are on, when they will let go their anchors and commence firing shells toward Vicksburg. No one, however, on this side is to fire until I burn two Coston signals (preparatory) and send up a rocket.

Thus, the preparation for the battle for Vicksburg where the Union forces finally prevailed in early July. *Red Rover* continued to take on the sick and the wounded, providing care for them, and providing medical supplies and other provisions to the other ships of the Squadron.

From the surrender of Vicksburg until the fall of 1864, *Red Rover*'s operational schedule was routine. She continued to ply the various rivers, providing medical assistance and provisions wherever needed. Based on periodic reports sent by Admiral Porter the Secretary of the Navy Welles, *Red Rover* was above Vicksburg on June 1, 1862, at Vicksburg July 1, at Memphis on August 1, and at Cairo December 1. Entries of January 15 and

February 15 indicate that she was still at Cairo but was under repairs. Acting Master Wm. Wells remained her commanding officer. On March 11, Fleet Captain Pennock reported: "The Red Rover came off the ways yesterday. The repairs upon her have been quite extensive and she will not be ready for ten or twelve days yet...."

Acting Volunteer Lieutenant Wells, U.S. Navy, commanding *U.S.S. Red Rover*, on May 11, provided the names of those received from the U.S.S. Covington to Lieutenant-Commander K.R. Breese:

> Sir: In obedience to your orders date May 9, this day received, I have the honor to report to you that I have received on board this ship from the U.S.S Covington John [T.] English [acting] third assistant engineer; S.C. Tarbell, paymaster's clerk; Michael Roach, seaman; Jacob S. Levier, seaman; Charles Barnett, seaman; Henry Lyons, first-class boy; Jacob Campbell, first-class boy; Eugene Sheftall, seaman; James Sullivan, seaman. From the U.S.S. Signal, John Galleger....

Fleet Captain Pennock reported to Admiral Porter, on March 15, in a general report that included other administrative items of business:

> ...Boggs writes from St. Louis that he is about shipping to this place two barges of ice, one containing 375 tons and the other 408 tons. The former is for the Red Rover, and the larger one I will send to you the best way I can. The cattle, he says, will be sent to you by the steamer Constitution.

Pennock apparently had some problems with the repairs of the *Red Rover*. On March 23, he wrote, "...I have been very anxious to get the Hastings and Red Rover finished, but, with all my grumbling and growling, fear they will not be ready to leave before the 2d or 3d of next month."

Red Rover must have finished her repairs, however, as W. Ferguson, Acting Master, Commanding *U.S.S. Silver Cloud* sent the following enclosure to LCdr T. Pattison, USN Commandant, Naval Station Memphis,

Tenn. on April 14, 1864. Though lengthy it provides an picture of the struggles endured, even late in the War:

SIR: I have the honor to report that in obedience to your order of the 12th instant I was taken in tow by the steamer Platte Valley and proceeded with all haste possible up the river to render assistance to our forces at Fort Pillow. About 20 miles above Memphis I spoke a steamer coming down and learned that Fort Pillow was captured by the rebels at 3 p. m. of the 12th. At 10:30 p. m. I had my fire walls repaired and steam up, but still continued lashed to the Platte Valley, as by that means I could make more haste. I arrived at Fulton, 3 miles below Fort Pillow, about 6 a. m. on the 13th and cast off from the Platte Valley, directing her to follow me up cautiously. At Fulton I learned that the rebel pickets were about one-half mile farther on. I soon came upon their outpost and commenced to shell the woods and hills in suspicious places, continuing to do so until I arrived opposite Fort Pillow. Although I could see parties of their cavalry moving about upon the hills, they did not return my fire. I rounded to a short distance above the fort and stood down the river close to the bank. All the buildings round the fort and the fort itself were on fire, and when I arrived abreast the fort several of our troops, some of them wounded, came out from their hiding places. I landed and took them on board and whilst doing so was fired upon by sharpshooters, but no person was injured. I then stood out in the river again and commenced to shell the hills. About this time some cavalry showed themselves on the hills with a flag of truce. I ceased firing and sent my cutter on shore in answer to it. The officer bearing the flag of truce had a proposal from General Forrest (a copy of which I forward) that he would give us possession of the fort and the country around it until 5 p. m. (it was then 8 a.m.) for the purpose of burying our dead and removing our wounded, who were suffering terribly from want of attention, provided I would acknowledge the parole of the wounded lying on the battle field. I agreed to his terms, and immediately made preparations for bringing down the wounded and burying our dead. The wounded I placed on board the Platte Valley for transportation to the New Madrid Hospital. I sent my surgeon in charge of them. Details of rebel soldiers and several of our soldiers on board the Platte Valley assisted my crew in bringing down the wounded, etc. In the meantime the U.S.S. New Era came down the river and sent a party on shore. After the Platte Valley had stood up the river with all the wounded found in the fort and around on the contested ground some 20 more came in from the rebel lines badly wounded. These were received by Fleet Surgeon Pinkney on board the Red Rover, which vessel fortunately came down the river at this time. The dead we buried amounted to about 150. We removed 69 wounded from the battle field, besides 20 I took on board before the flag of truce was sent in by the enemy. ....

Writing from off Fort Pillow, April 13, 1864 at 6 p. m., N.D. Wetmore, Jr provided the following account to the editors of *Argus Magazine*:

Editors, Argus:

Gentlemen: The combined forces (numbering between 7,000 and 8,000) of Major-General Forrest, General Chalmers, Colonel McCulloch, and Colonel Bell, the two latter commanding brigades, made an assault upon our fortifications at about 6 a. m. on yesterday. Our force consisted of about 250 whites and 350 blacks. The U.S.S. New Era, Acting Master James Marshall commanding, lying off the fort, shelled the rebels and drove them from a position which they had gained on the south side of the fort. They again assaulted our works from the north side. Owing to the dense timber, it was impossible to dislodge them, although Captain Marshall kept a continual shower of shell and shrapnel raining down upon them; but so small was the force in the garrison and so overwhelming the rebel force, that at about 3:30 p. m. the enemy carried our works and the gallant few which were left [were] taken prisoners. The guns of the fort consisted of two 12-pounder howitzers, two 10-pounder rifled, and two 10-pounder Parrotts, six pieces in all. Major Booth and two captains of the Sixth United States Artillery (colored) were killed early in the engagement, also two lieutenants of same command badly wounded. Of the Thirteenth Tennessee Cavalry, Captains Bradford, Porter, and Leaming, also Lieutenant Barr and some others, who could not be identified. Major Bradford was taken prisoner, and reported by the rebels as having been paroled the liberty of their camp, and having violated it by escaping during last night, but I was told that he was taken out by the rebels late last evening and shot. Captain Young, provost-marshal of post, taken a prisoner and paroled the liberty of their camp, says that our forces behaved gallantly throughout the whole action; that our loss in killed will exceed 200; he also stated that General Forrest shot one of his own command for refusing quarters to our men. Lieutenant-Commander Thomas Pattison, commandant of station at Memphis, receiving dispatches at 7 p. m. last evening from the commanding officer of New Era that he was nearly out of ammunition, ordered the mail steamer Platte Valley to take in tow U.S.S. Silver Cloud, Acting Master W. Ferguson, commanding, and proceed at once to the scene of action. The boilers of the Silver Cloud being at the time down, through the energy of Captain Ferguson, in three hours they were up, and by 12 [had] steam enough to make 6 knots against the current. The two boats kept together until 2 a.m., when Captain Ferguson ordered Captain Riley, commanding Platte Valley, to drop astern. At 7 a. m. we arrived in sight of Fort Pillow. The commissary and other public buildings, together with some 12 stores, private property, were in flames. The rebels could be seen moving about applying torches to the barracks, huts, and stables. Captain Ferguson ordered his pilot to move up within range for 5-second shells. For some thirty minutes or more he continued throwing shell and shrapnel at detached squads as they moved about. The cannon, which was mounted on field carriage, the rebels had moved during the night from the fort to their outposts. A flag of truce appearing, Captain Ferguson ordered his men to cease firing, and answered it by sending a small boat with an officer and 6 men to the shore. Presently it returned with a communication from Major-General Forrest, saying that a large number of our wounded were suffering for the want of proper attention, saying that in the event certain stipulations (which he mentioned) were agreed to, that he would withdraw his forces to the outer works and give him possession of the fort until 5 p.m., occupying same under flag of truce for the purpose of burying the dead and removing the wounded. Captain Ferguson, knowing that the shells from his guns would necessarily explode among our wounded, causing a still greater loss of life to us, entered into an agreement with Major Charles W. Anderson, aid-de-camp to General Forrest, and acting under his authority, the purport of which was that on our part we would not disturb their men while gathering the small arms nor allow anything whatever to be removed from the battle field. On their part they were to allow us to land as many men as we might deem necessary to bury the dead and take the wounded off, they requiring one hour to withdraw their remaining armed forces to the outworks. At about 12 m. we commenced. Captain Ferguson signaled the Platte Valley to move up and come alongside, which she did do, and the wounded, some fifty-odd, placed on board. A list of their names I herewith append. The rebels rendered us efficient aid, facilitating as much as possible getting the wounded on board transport. Those wounded who could walk were generally brought down the bluffs, supported on either side by a rebel soldier. Too much praise can not be bestowed upon Captain Riley, as well as all other officers of the Platte Valley, for the manner in which they provided for the wounded, requiring the passengers to give up their staterooms, furnishing at once proper sustenance of food, and nourishing drinks to those who were unable to eat. There were a great many ladies on board who, God bless them, true to their nature, went at once to work alleviating as far as possible their sufferings. After the Platte Valley left, some 12 to 15 wounded were sent in from the Confederate camp. The United States naval hospital boat Red Rover landed, and Fleet Surgeon Ninian Pinkney, with his usual promptness, provided comfortable quarters for them, and with his little army of assistant surgeons soon had their wounds dressed. The names of those taken charge of by Surgeon Pinckney I did not get, the accompanying list being the names only of those sent to Cairo. Now that the excitement is over, the thought of those charred bodies, together with the nausea occasioned by the burning human flesh, and the 200 or more dead bodies mangled, dying as they did, pleading for quarter, many with faces distorted with pain, eyes bayoneted, skulls broken, and some with bowels torn from the human casements, some so besmeared with blood and the flesh of comrades as to render them incog. to even their own fathers and mothers, it has so sickened me that I can write no more. Messrs. editors, I must add that in storming a fort where such desperate resistance is offered, that many, very many, must fall; but at Fort Pillow I have every evidence that instead of honorable warfare that the Confederates pursued that of indiscriminate butchery.

On April 19, Rear-Admiral Porter, detached Acting Ensign Charles King, U.S. Navy, from the *Red Rover* and sent him to the command of U.S.S. Little Rebel: "Sir: You are hereby detached from the U.S.S. Red Rover, and you will report to the commanding officer of the U.S.S. Little Rebel for duty and command of that vessel."

At the time *Red Rover* was at the mouth of the Red River and it appears that King may not have ever left the hospital ship. Memphis came under attack by the Confederates on August 22, 1864, and reports indicate that *Red Rover* was there at the time. In reports from Admiral Porter to Secretary of the Navy Welles, which state the locations of the ships, Acting Ensign Charles King is listed as commanding officer of *Red Rover* May 21, September 8, and October 15. The location of the ship on those dates is not given. In the report of November 15, King and *Red Rover* are at New Orleans and on December 1 they are at Memphis.

Even as the end of the war neared administration continued to be an issue. In a report of Acting Rear-Admiral Lee regarding appointment and pay of pilots wrote the Secretary of the Navy from the Flagship Black Hawk at New Orleans, La., January 30, 1865.

SIR: The Department's communication of 23d of November, enquiring whether Western pilots are appointed as pilots in the naval service and sworn in or hired temporarily, was duly received. The pressure of duty in connection with Army operations at that time, and separation from my files, prevented my giving the subject prompt attention. I have issued a call for exact information on the subject, and meanwhile I have the honor to inform the Department that the majority of the pilots employed in this squadron are appointed by the commander-in-chief and sworn in; some are hired temporarily and receive the same pay as appointed pilots. I enclose a petition signed by 28 of the appointed first-class pilots of this squadron for an increase of the present pay, from $250 to $300 per month, which last sum they state was the rate of pay established early in the war by General Grant's order for pilots on Army transports, which they still receive, while pilots in the merchant service, receive from $450 to $750 per month, and that at the present rates of pay, few good pilots are willing to enter the naval service, thus necessitating the employment of incompetent men or causing pecuniary loss to those of ability and experience. I recommend this increase of pay to the favorable consideration of the Department both as just and economical. It has been customary to draft them from the pilot's associations, or impress them summarily, for temporary service from boats plying on the river, and, as trade is increasing, the difficulty of getting pilots by arbitrary means will be greatly increased. I am informed that the provost-marshal at St. Louis decides that a pilot is not excused from the draft because he is at the time a pilot in the Navy. It is difficult to get pilots, and a great misapplication of them, to put them in the ranks of the Army. I recommend that it be made the duty of all provost-marshals promptly to turn over to the commanding officer of this squadron, through the commandant of the naval station at Mound City, all the pilots for the Western waters who are legally drafted for military service in the Army.

[Enclosure.]

U.S. Mississippi SQUADRON, November 26, 1864.

Sir: The undersigned, pilots in the U.S. Mississippi Squadron, respectfully call your attention to the fact that for a long time past the wages of pilots in the merchant service and army transports have been in excess of what we receive in the squadron.

Early in this year the wages of pilots on army transports and the Mississippi Marine Brigade were (by order of General Grant) established at $300 per month, and every pilot working on army transport is receiving that money, while pilots in the merchant service are receiving much more—say, from $450 to as much as

$750 per month.

At the present rate of wages few good pilots are willing to enter the service, thus forcing the employment of incompetent and inexperienced men to fill vacancies, to the great detriment of the service, besides making the duties of competent men more arduous.

Many of us have been in the service a long time. A few, from the first organization of a naval force on these waters, and we do not desire to leave the service, but we do think our willingness to serve our country should not be made a matter of so much pecuniary loss to ourselves.

We therefore respectfully request that the wages of first-class pilots in the Mississippi Squadron be $300 per month.

Hoping for your favorable consideration of our request, we are, very respectfully,
    your obedient servants
    GEORGE B. FOWLER,
    First-Class Pilot.
    E.L. WILKENSON,
    First-Class Pilot.
    JOSEPH M. CHAMMANTS,
    First Pilot.
    W.M. ATTENBOROUGH,
    U.S.S. Essex, First-Class Pilot.
    D.A. HINER,
    U.S.S. General Lyon, First Pilot.
    J.C. WOODRUFF,
    U.S.S. Red Rover, First Pilot

Reporting in July 1865 from the Flagship *Tempset*, Mound City to Secretary Welles, Fleet Captain Bryson, included in the disposition of vessels of the Mississippi Squadron: "Sir: The following is the present disposition of the vessels of this squadron. ...In temporary use.—Red Rover, hospital; General Lyon, Samson, Dahlia, Hyacinth, Laurel, Myrtle, Thistle, tugs."

As the post-war wind down occurred Acting Rear-Admiral Lee, U.S. Navy, provided to the Chief of Bureau of Navigation and Office of Detail a list of officers transferred with the U.S.S. *Red Rover*. From Mound City he wrote on August 12, 1865:

Sir: I have this day transferred to Commodore John W.. Livingston the U.S.S. Red Rover (hospital vessel), with her officers and crew. Below is the list of the officers:

A. W. Pearson, acting assistant paymaster; J. J. Irwin, acting ensign; William Sprague, acting first assistant engineer; M. L. Gerould, acting assisting surgeon; R.G. VanNess, acting master's mate; Benjamin Nelson, acting master's mate; Thomas Finnie, acting second assistant engineer; Thomas McAllister, acting third assistant engineer; F.M. McCord, acting master's mate; C. S. Scanlan, acting master's mate; John C. Farnsworth, paymaster's clerk.

From the Flagship *Tempest* on the Mississippi River, August 12, 1865, the report of Acting Rear-Admiral Lee to the Secretary of the Navy Welles, gave disposition of remaining vessels of the Mississippi Squadron and proposed to haul down his flag: "Sir: In conformity with the Department's orders of 29th July, I have, after putting out of commission the vessels of this squadron intended for sale and turning them over to Commodore Livingston, issued orders for turning over to him the remaining vessels, the Tempest, Kate, and Volunteer, and the hospital ship Red Rover. My flag will be hauled down on the 14th instant.. My address will be Washington, D.C."

Acting Rear Admiral Samuel Phillips Lee (February 13, 1812-June 5, 1897) had assumed command of the Squadron on November 1, 1864. Lee, from the distinguished Lee family of Virginia, was the son of Francis Lightfoot and Jane Fitzgerald Lee, the grandson of Richard Henry Lee, and the great nephew of Richard Lightfoot Lee. Appointed a midshipman in the Navy November 22, 1825, Lee served in various capacities from then until the outbreak of the Civil War. Early in the war he, as commander of the *Oneida*, participated in the attack on New Orleans and at Vicksburg under Farragut. In September 1862, just after his promotion to captain, Lee was appointed an acting rear admiral and given command of the North Atlantic

Blockading Squadron, then operating off the coast of Virginia and North Carolina. In 1864, when an attack of Wilmington was contemplated, Secretary of the Navy Welles removed him because he did not consider him to be a fighting admiral or a man of prompt action. Sent to command the Mississippi Squadron, Admiral Lee seems to have done very good work on the Cumberland and Tennessee Rivers. Lee retired from the Navy in 1873, spent his final years in Washington, D.C., dying at Silver Springs, MD, of a stroke of paralysis. Admiral Lee was never a popular hero but seems to have been one of the most conscientious and efficient officers of his time. He was relieved in August, 1865, by Commodore John W. Livingston who closed up the affairs of the Mississippi Squadron in November, 1865.

The *Red Rover* continued to care for Navy patients throughout this period until November 17, 1865, when her eleven remaining patients were transferred to the steamer *Grampus*. During her career she had admitted only three less than 2,500 patients; 1,697 had been admitted during June 11,1862 to March 31,1865, 332 being from Southern States, 343 from Northern States, 231 from Western States, 376 born in foreign countries, and the nativity of 415 not ascertained. Out of the 1,697 patients admitted, 157 died. An additional 780 patients were cared for by the *Red Rover* during the period April 1 to November 17, 1865. Her last record of those employed in her medical department is dated April 30, 1865. Sister M. Veronica and Sister Adela were still on board and it is presumed they remained until November 17, 1865, the last day of the ship's service. Dr. George H. Bixby, who had contributed so much to the effectiveness of the hospital ship, was honorably discharged from the Navy on September 26, 1865. He resumed his medical practice in Boston where he engaged in important research and wrote numerous treatises. Dr Hopkins went on to similar fame in his own field.

Stripped of her gun and iron plate, the *Red Rover* was sold at public auction in Mound City by Solomon A. Silver on November 29,1865. Her purchaser was A. M. Carpenter who paid $4,500 for the hulk of the first United States Navy Hospital Ship.

****

APPENDIX A

Statistical Data

U.S.S. RED ROVER. Acquisition. — Captured; purchased from Illinois prize court September 30, 1862, by Navy Department. Cost.—$10,000. Description.— Class: Side-wheel steamer; wood. Rate: 4th. Tonnage.—786. Draft.—Deeply laden, 8'. Speed—Upstream, 9 knots. Engines—Two. Diameter of cylinder, 28"; stroke, 5'. Boilers.—Five. Battery.—September 2, 1863, 1 32- pdr. 33 cwt; August 7, 1805, similar to the preceding. Disposition.—Sold at public auction, November 29, 1865, at Mound City, Ill., by Solomon A. Silver, to A. M. Carpenter, for $4,500. Remarks.—Commissioned December 26, 1862, at Cairo, Ill.

APPENDIX B

Officers of Navy Yards, Shore Stations, and Vessels, 1 January 1865 Mississippi Squadron:

Acting Rear-Admiral Samuel P. Lee, Commanding.
Staff: Lieutenant Commander C. A. Babcock, Acting Fleet Captain.
Lieutenant F. J. Naile, Flag Lieutenant.
Acting Volunteer Lieutenant, Wm. G. Saltonstall.
Surgeon Ninian Pinkney, Fleet Surgeon.
Paymaster Ed. T. Dunn, Fleet Paymaster.
Acting Chief Engineer Samuel Bickerstaff, Fleet Engineer.
Acting Master, C. R. Knowles.
Acting Ensigns, Wm. Ringgold Cooper and C. C. Cushing.

HOSPITAL SHIP *RED ROVER*.

Acting Ensign, Charles King.
Fleet Surgeon, Ninian Pinkney.
Passed Assistant Surgeon, J. S. Knight.
Acting Assistant Surgeons, George H. Bixby and J. T. Field.
Acting Assistant Paymaster, Alexander W. Pearson.
Acting Ensign, J. J. Irwin.
Acting Master's Mate, R. G. Van Ness.
Engineers: Acting Chief, William T. Buffinton; Acting First Assistant, William Sprague; Acting Second Assistant, Wm. M. Fletcher; Acting Third Assistants, William H. Vanwert and J. T. English.
Acting Carpenter, Harlow Kinney.

MOUND CITY, ILLINOIS. NAVAL STATION.

Commodore, John W. Livingston.
Commander, Aaron K. Hughes.
Acting Volunteer Lieutenant, Peter O'Kell.

Acting Master, Daniel C. Bower.
Acting Ensigns, James M. Bailey and Frank Sherman.
Acting Master's Mate, Robert B. Moore.
Surgeon, Wm. T. Hord.
Acting Assistant Surgeon, Vincent H. Gaskill.
Paymasters, C. C. Jackson and A. H. Gilman.
Assistant Paymaster, Geo. W. Beaman.
Acting Assistant Paymaster, James F. Hamilton.
Engineers: Acting Chief, James B. Fulton; Acting Second Assistant, Richard Fengler.Acting Boatswain, Wm. Allen.
Acting Gunner, Asa P. Snyder.
Sailmaker, Wm. N. Maull.

APPENDIX C

A listing of the women who served with the *Red Rover* while it was a part of the Army's Western Gunboat Flotilla and after she became a part of the U.S. Navy's Mississippi Squadron.

NAME	SERVED AS	WITH	FROM	TO
Sister Adela	Nurse	Army and	06-01-62	03-31-65
	Sister of Holy Cross	Navy		
Sister Veronica	Nurse	Army and	06-01-62	08-01-65
	Sister of Holy Cross	Navy		
Sister Calista	Nurse	Navy	12-01-62	02-28-63
	Sister of Holy Cross			
Sister St John	Nurse	Navy	02-21-62	09-30-63
	Sister of Holy Cross			
Ellen Campbell	Nurse	Navy	09-01-63	03-26-63
Georgina Harris	Nurse	Navy	07-01-63	09-26-63
Sarah Nothing	Nurse	Navy	12-01-63	06-15-64
Betsy Young	Nurse	Navy	09-01-63	08-20-65
Ann Stokes	Nurse	Navy	01-25-63	05-31-64
	Contraband	Navy	06-01-64	10-25-64
Ann Graves	Chambermaid	Army	04-13-62	08-31-62
Mary Warfield	Chambermaid	Army	05-22-62	08-31-62
Betsy Bishop	Laundress	Army	08-01-62	09-30-62
Mary Bryant	Laundress	Army	06-08-62	09-30-62
Marie Cassidy	Laundress	Army	06-21-62	08-31-62
Eliza McLothia	Laundress	Army	06-27-62	07-31-62
Mattie Perkins	Laundress	Army	08-01-62	09-30-62
Nancy Rogers	Laundress	Army	08-01-62	09-30-62
Sarah Watson	Laundress	Army	09-17-62	09-30-62
Nancy Buell	Laundress	Navy	09-021-63	10-26-63
Sallie Bohannon	Laundress	Navy	09-01-63	11-23-63
Mary Dalton	Laundress	Navy	02-21-63	08-31-65
Mary Ann Donald	Laundress	Navy	10-24-64	11-23-64
Lucinda Jenkins	Laundress	Navy	01-01-64	06-13-64
Alice Kennedy	Laundress	Navy	01-01-63	07-16-63
Sarah Kinno	Laundress	Navy	02-13-64	??-25-63
Alice McLean	Laundress	Navy	01-01-64	03-24-64
Sabra Miller	Laundress	Navy	01-01-64	03-26-64
Ann Ragan	Laundress	Navy	10-24-64	11-23-64
Adelia Robertson	Laundress	Navy	07-01-64	10-25-64
Margaret Jackson	Contraband	Navy	05-10-63	10-04-64
Eliza Owens	Contraband	Navy	01-26-63	04-30-63

APPENDIX D

Photographs

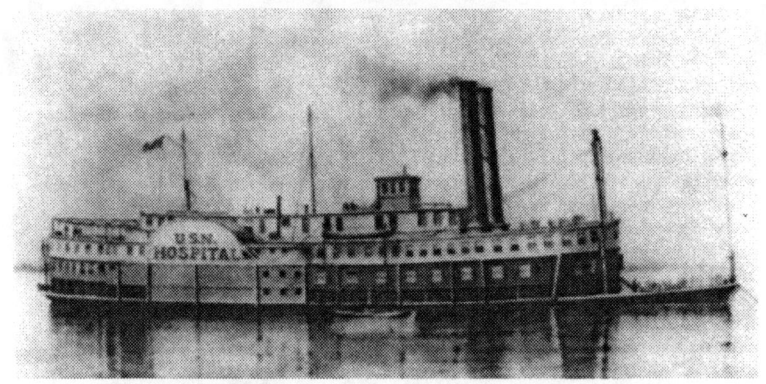

U.S.S. Red Rover, Naval Hospital Ship 1862-1865

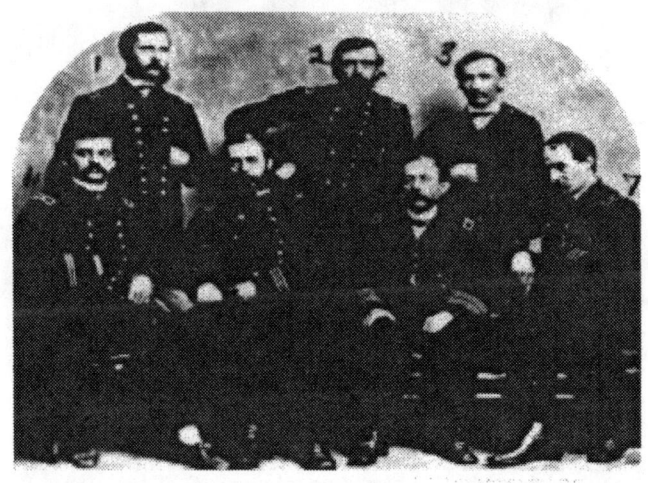

Medical officers of the *Red Rover*. Standing left to right: Jacob T. Field, A.W. Pearson, George Lawrence. Sitting left to right: George H. Bixby, James S. Knight, Ninian Pinkney and Michael Bradley. Other medical officers who served aboard the hospital ship were George H. Hopkins, J. B. Parker, William F. McNutt and William H. Willson.

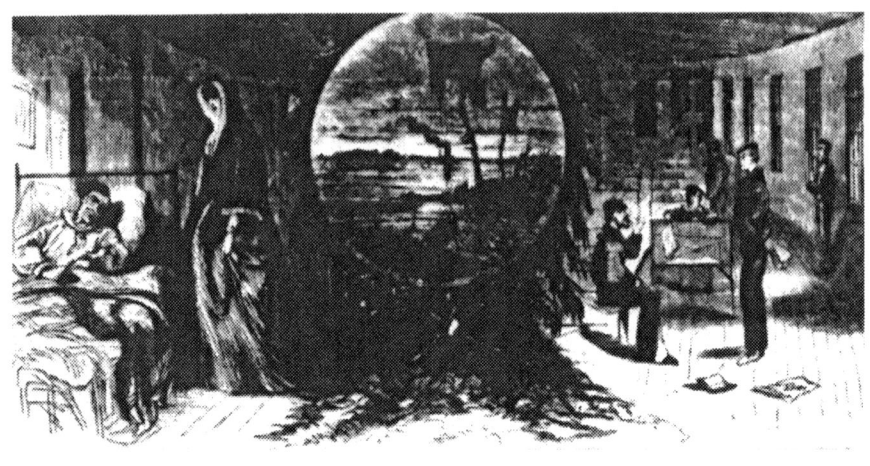

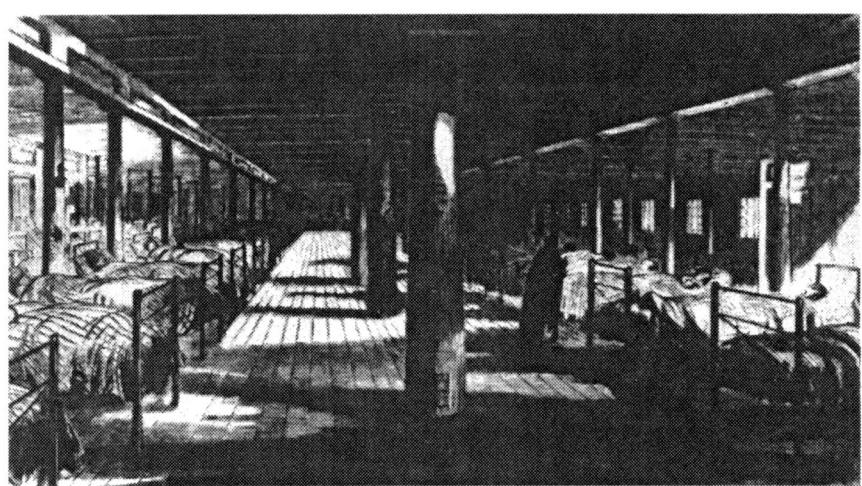

Two of the three photographs that appeared in *Harper's Weekly*, May 9, 1863. The third is one of *Red Rover*, which is very similar but not identical to the one above.

BIBLIOGRAPHY

All Hands Magazine, February 1962, pps 59-63.

Civil War History, June 1998; FindArticles.com, located at http:www/ findarticle.com

"C.S. Steamer *Red Rover*" by Brian M. Green, *Society of Philatelic American Journal*, Volume 40, No. 10, June 1978, pps 679-680.

Dictionary of American Biography, Scribners and Co. NY, 1936.

Dictionary of American Fighting Ships, Vol. 7.

Harper's Weekly, May 9, 1863, a full page of illustrations of the *Red Rover*.

"Holy Cross Sisters 1st Navy Nurses" by Sister M. John Francis, Jacksonville (IL) Courier, December 23, 1962.

Missouri Historical Review, Vol LX, Oct 1965, No. 1, pgs 31-49. "A History of the First U.S. Navy Hospital Ship" by Edward C Kenney.

Navy Department, Bureau of Medicine and Surgery, Letters, 1861-1865.

Navy Department, Officers Letters, 1861-1865.

Navy Department. Letters and reports of officers of the western Flotilla, later transferred to Navy and redesignated Mississippi Squadron, 1861-1865.

"On the King's Highway: A History of the Sisters of the Holy Cross of St. Mary of the Immaculate Conception," by Sister Mary Eleanor; D. Appleton, New York, 1931.

Scientific American. New Series, Volume 6, Issue 16:, pg 242: [dated April 19, 1862]

Scientific American. New Series, Volume 6, Issue 17: [dated April 26, 1862], pgs 257-272 ; *Red Rover*, pg 259

U.S. Naval Institute Proceedings, Nov 1968, "*Red Rover*: First Hospital Ship of the U.S. Navy" by W. T. Adams, pg 149-151.

USS *Red Rover*, Ship's Deck Log, December 26, 1862-January 1,1865.

USS *Red Rover*, Medical Journals, June 10. 1862-November 17, 1865.

USS *Red Rover*, Muster Rolls, August, 1863-April 1865.

USS *Red Rover*, Abstract of Patients, June 10, 1862-November 17, 1865.

USS *Red Rover*, Ledger of "Deaths-Invoices Receipts & C," June 10, 1862-November 17, 1865.

War Department. Extracts from (Army) Hospital muster rolls and pay records of Nurses, Matrons and Attendants, 1861-1865.

Official Records of the Union and Confederate Navies in the War of the Rebellion (Washington, D.C., 1898-1922), 10 volumes.

Official Records of the Union and Confederate Armies in the War of the Rebellion (Washington, D.C., 1880-1602), 130 volumes.

Series I - Volume 18: West Gulf Blockading Squadron (February 21, 1862 - July 14, 1862).

Series I - Volume 19: West Gulf Blockading Squadron (July 15, 1862 - March 14, 1863).

Series I - Volume 22: West Gulf Blockading Squadron (January 1, 1865 - January 31, 1866); Naval Forces on Western Waters (May 8, 1861 - April 11, 1862).

Series I - Volume 23: Naval Forces on Western Waters (April 12, 1862 - December 31, 1862).

Series I - Volume 24: Naval Forces on Western Waters (January 1, 1863 - May 17, 1863).

Series I - Volume 25: Naval Forces on Western Waters (May 18, 1863 - February 29, 1864).

Series I - Volume 26: Naval Forces on Western Waters (March 1, 1864 - December 31, 1864).

Series I - Volume 27: Naval Forces on Western Waters (January 1, 1865 - September 6, 1865); Supply Vessels (January 1, 1865 - September 6, 1865).

Series I - Volume 7: North Atlantic Blockading Squadron (March 8, 1862 - September 4, 1862).

Series II - Volume 1: Statistical Data of Union and Confederate Ships; Muster Roles of Confederate Government Vessels; Letters of Marque and Reprisals; Confederate Department Investigations.

The war of the rebellion: a compilation of the official records of the Union and Confederate armies. / Series 1 - Volume 39 (Part III).

The war of the rebellion: a compilation of the official records of the Union and Confederate armies. / Series 1 - Volume 8.

The war of the rebellion: a compilation of the official records of the Union and Confederate armies. / Series 2 - Volume 4.

The war of the rebellion: a compilation of the official records of the Union and Confederate armies. / Series 3 - Volume 2.

The war of the rebellion: a compilation of the official records of the Union and Confederate armies. / Series 3 - Volume 5.

The war of the rebellion: a compilation of the official records of the Union and Confederate armies. / Series 4 - Volume 4

Printed in the United States
63119LVS00003B/288